My Burpee's Shadow

Inspiring Stories About Embracing Fitness

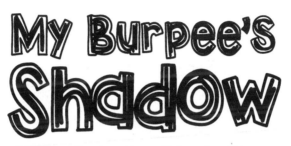

My Burpee's Shadow

Inspiring Stories About Embracing Fitness

Written and Illustrated by

Robby Wagner

Edited by

Kelly Haught

To Romeo (my dog), My Friends and My Fitness Family:
You All Mean the World to Me.

Table of Contents

<u>Acknowledgement</u>

First, I would like to give a big thanks to my fitness family, new and old, for supporting me in writing this book and for continuing to bless me with your love and friendship each and every day. I'm deeply grateful for every single one of you. I look forward to the future as we change the world together.

I would like to thank all who have supported me throughout my comedy career and to the many who have cheered me on as I grew into new areas of the entertainment industry.

I'd like to give a special thanks to my Editor and amazing friend, Kelly Haught, for all the hard work and time put in to make this book so wonderful. Nobody else could've done what you've done and I'm not sure this book would have ever been finished without all of your help and support. I'm truly grateful for you and all you've done to make this book happen.

I'd like to thank my mom, Patty Porter, for giving me the love and strength that I needed to carry on through life on my own. This book, as well as my entire career, would not have been possible without your love. I miss you everyday but you're still alive in my heart. Thank you for always being passionate about loving me and making sure I knew it. I think about it every day.

Last but not least, I'd like to thank God for always being close by when I thought I was alone in this world. Thank you for the talents you've given me and the many people you've blessed me with over the years through friendships.

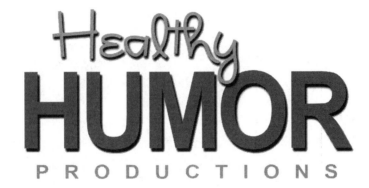

The Warm-up

Hello, Class!

Thank you for deciding to read *My Burpee's Shadow*. This book, while not a class, is set up like one of my typical bootcamp classes. There is the *warm-up*, the *workout*, a *group challenge*, and the *cool-down*.

This is not your typical fitness book and it certainly isn't an instruction manual. The purpose is to share different peoples' stories about their lives before and after starting an exercise regimen, starting with mine. Throughout the book, there'll be moments of seriousness, humor, and motivation.

I noticed a broad variety of people who take my class, and so decided to explore deeper by inviting everyone to share their personal story. What were their lives like before exercising and how are they better now? I'm very pleased with the responses of those who wanted to be a part in sharing with the world their own personal journeys into fitness. Even though nutrition plays a huge part of our wellness, these stories focus much more on exercise and our personal reasons to begin working out.

The Burpee Shadow

To understand the title of this book, it may help to know what a burpee is. Is it how a toddler tries to say *burp*? No. Well, maybe. But, in this case, no! The burpee is actually named after a physiologist by the name of Royal H. Burpee who developed a 4-part combination exercise in 1940 as part of a test to gauge fitness. Burpees are also known as up-downs to some people, even though up-down-ups would be a more accurate description. Or, to some, up-down-up-then-throw up might be a more suitable description. Whichever way, the most popular way fitness classes perform them are: squat down, jump back into a plank, do a push-up, jump back forward to squat position, and jump up when coming back up to start position. And just like people, there are all different types and variations of the burpee available.

The *burpee* used in the title is a representation of the amazing people in this book and hopefully you, *too*...whether now or in the future. It represents the people of this book in the *now*. A burpee is a difficult exercise to perform: it can often times take a while to get good at. For some, it's the result of hard work, dedication, sweat, and motivation. For others, it may be as simple as starting to do them again after years without. Whatever has brought them to the burpee, or continuous and rigorous training, the metaphor is that everyone came from somewhere and is now in this circle together. We do them according to what our bodies are capable of doing and we are getting better each day, each workout.

The *shadow* of the burpee represents our past. We all have one that is unique and different from the next person. The shadow is a reminder of where we came from and it will always be attached to us. However, it is vital to remember that it is always underneath or to the side of us when we move. We can also choose to stand in full light, surrounded from all angles, so our shadow becomes lighter...almost nonexistent to the eye. When we choose to do our burpees, our shadow has no choice but to follow and participate. We can see our shadow, or past, imitate the strength we are bringing to our present when we choose to be active in exercise. The shadow can't move forward on it's own, but when we work to better ourselves, in the present, the results are positive not only for us now, but for our future shadows, as well.

The Workout

Let's get started. Most people see me as a fitness junkie. They see the *now* version of me, but what most people don't know is where it all began. I'm no different than most people and at times may be a bit more extreme in the bad choices I've made throughout my years growing up, as well as an adult. I've contemplated many times if I'm the right person to lead so many people in their own health journeys each and every day. After all, I spent my entire childhood overweight. I've had several failed relationships (marriages included): I smoked (tobacco and a few times something a little greener): I drank regularly for fun, and my past is littered with many unhealthy lose-weight-fast diets. Even though these are all bad things, sharing them is essential to reach many people who think that it's too late to become healthy and make big changes in their lives. Now, when the question, *Am I the right person to lead so many people in their fitness journeys* comes up, the answer is, *yes*! Of course, I am. Who better to help create change in others than someone who has already created a huge change in himself?

Why I Work Out

I don't feel that the reasons *why* we start working out are as important as the fact that we *are* working out. That being said, the need for change can be a powerful force. I needed big change in my life. I grew up overweight and at a fat 17 years old, I encountered one of the hardest things in my life: I suddenly lost my healthy mom to countless strokes that left her speechless and paralyzed over the next decade. In that heartbreaking process, I lost my family, whom I was once close with, altogether.

My girlfriend at the time blatantly informed me that she had cheated on me with another guy during this depressing time in my life.

It wasn't until I found myself in tears, raging in the midst of what looked like a bomb explosion in my room, screaming at the top of my lungs at my own reflection in my dark bedroom window, all while pressing a knife to my throat, that I actually felt a need to live. As crazy as it sounds, that blind and raging moment provided the exact clarity I needed to help me design the person I am today. It was in that one fork-in-the-road moment that I decided to make myself strong and conquer anything life was going to put in front of me. I needed to change... and so I did.

I went on to lose 85lbs in what seemed to happen overnight (it was in reality about 3 months). I needed to be different and look different. It was time to leave the old and weak Robby behind and become anew. I shaved my head and started researching at the bookstore how to lose weight. I came across a theory that would be my biggest influence on fitness from a book I found about my childhood hero, Bruce Lee. His notes, consisting of his diet and his thoughts and how-to exercise regimen were compiled into this book. As I applied Bruce Lee's theories, they literally changed my life. His mindset is my foundation. I still religiously use it today as my personal program, as well as in any principles I teach.

Looking back at this unique period of my life, after this incredible weight loss at the age of 18, I realize that even though I had physically changed who I was, I still had all the same emotional problems going on inside of me. Not only were they fresh in my life at that point, they would continue to force me to fight for my overall well-being, like an ongoing battle of good vs. evil. Everything I had at the time was now lost: a healthy mom and best friend, my relationship with my family, my girlfriend, and to top it off, my welcome stay at my mom's home after my evil stepfather figure kicked me out to move in his adult son. I felt completely lost in the world, alone, and completely powerless. I truly believe that exercise was the stepping stone for my emotional and mental health. By choosing this positive route for my body, the process of becoming physically stronger seemed to automatically adopt other positive decisions in time. My own experience with exercise has been an unending journey and great outlet for me that helped me stay high when I was so tempted to fall low. While the outside of me was strong and the inside was not, I believe that because of exercise, the strong part of me overtook the weak side in my life.

All throughout my adult life, exercise has been my method of empowering myself. It has always served to give me confidence, relieve stresses, and make me a happier and more productive person. I find that the standard I hold myself to when I exercise in a gym, at a park, or at home transcends into everything else that I do in my everyday life. I'm a better friend, a harder worker, a kinder stranger, and just a better person overall.

Everyone needs exercise. And everyone will have their own unique reason why they exercise in the beginning. Some may seek vanity from it while others may seek more energy. There are countless possible reasons why we want to exercise but whatever that initial purpose is for each of us, the important thing is that it compels us to start. Your desired destinations may change throughout your life, but one of the vehicles that will help you get there will always remain constant – and that is to exercise.

Memories of a Fat Kid – The Life and Times of a Fat Little Robby

The following are a few stories of growing up as an overweight kid and some explanations and reasoning of who I am today. They span from grade school until high school and focus on some strengths and weaknesses I've had along the way. They are discoveries of myself as I look to my past and reflect on the trials I had as a fat little Robby.

The Truth of a Dad Man

My biological father has only had the privilege of meeting me three times in my life. He really is a mysterious person: I do not know him, where he is, or if he's even alive. Legend has it that he's had 24 kids by 100 different women. If so, I imagine how awesome it'd be to have 23 half brothers and sisters that are just like me. Maybe they're all fitness instructors, too, and one day we'll form our own gym. We could call it *24 Bastards Fitness*. People could join, and just like him, have no obligation or commitment to us whatsoever. They could even skip paying each month without any kind of repercussion. I doubt it'll happen but one can dream! I bring up this stranger in my life because I believe his presence – or rather, lack thereof, was the start of my entire negative outlook on myself growing up and continuing through part of my adult life.

My father stood a whopping 5'8" tall. He was a country western singer by night and last I remembered, went door-to-door to try and scrape up money by mowing peoples' lawns. He got women to fall in love with him and then lived off them until he found the next one who had more to offer. He was adopted from Guam and these are the only things I know about him. My mom never said a bad thing about him to me but she didn't have to because people have a way of revealing who they really are on their own.

By age 8 I was used to the names my dad would call me, his laughter after almost breaking my little fingers each day, and the lies he'd tell me for his own entertainment and joy. It was the end of summer before starting the 3rd grade when I had my third- and last, visit to see him. On this particular trip, he had much more in store for me than I was used to. I had started gaining a little weight that summer and that's what he decided to play on, alongside his current girlfriend and her daughter, who was a year older than I was. Each day, he'd remind me how fat I was and how much disbelief he held that my mom could raise such an ugly, fat boy. He had a natural,

7

raw talent for making people feel bad.

I remember this one particular time vividly. We went to the grocery store one afternoon. While we were checking out at the cashier, there was an obviously mentally handicapped boy running around, yelling and drooling all over the place, causing everyone to look. At that moment, my dad said, "Look, Robby! That's you in 3 years." I remember the cashier and a few people in line laughing at his comment. He then put his arms around his girlfriend's daughter and hugged her, saying to me, "Why can't you be thin and good looking like Marlena?"

This particular part of my life really played a big role in how I saw myself over the years to come. It was an unfortunate time, as well as a painfully long process to overcome, but in the end, I couldn't ask to be a better *me*.

Boobies Killed My Acting Career

A milestone in every fat boy's life is when they discover they have boobs. For me, that glorious day happened in 3rd grade while at the public pool. It was around that age when us boys discovered that we liked women's breasts. And little did I know, I had them! That's right, I had them and nobody else did. It wasn't until I took my shirt and bra off in front of my friends at the public pool that I knew I'd never go swimming again. They couldn't have laughed any harder without dying, and the insults born that day became their new favorite activity. I hated being the butt (and boob) of every hooter joke there was to be said in grade school.

I had to figure out how to handle this. So, I thought up a serious condition to tell the other kids about why I couldn't take my shirt off anymore. The condition I made up was very simple. Basically, my "doctor" told me that the sun burned me so badly that I could die if I was not wearing a shirt at all times outside. However, the sun was okay for my face, arms, legs, and feet. It was only critical in my chest, back, and belly area. This worked amongst my so-called *friends*, even though I am 100% island boy and the sun is one of my closest friends. They still made fun of me but at least I didn't have to show the perky round baby watermelons off anymore...because men can be real pigs, am I right?

That year, my aunt knew someone who was casting kids to be extras in the movie, *Rambo: First Blood Part II*, which was being filmed in my hometown, Yuma, Arizona. He told her to bring me down and I could be in it. After she told me about it, I talked it over with my agents, a.k.a. the voices in my head, and decided that it was a bad career move for me. I really wanted to meet Sylvester Stallone but I didn't want to be one of the child extras that had to jump up and down shirtless in the movie. I'm not sure if that's what the part was but that's all I could imagine, and I definitely wasn't about to take any chances.

I kept imagining Sly saying in his Rocky Balboa voice, "Hey Pauly! Why does the kid have boobs? Get him out of here, it's not a *girly* movie, ya know?" (Hopefully, you read that in your best Sylvester Stallone voice.)

Throughout the rest of my childhood and into my teen years, I managed to keep my cantaloupes hidden from most of the world. I was embarrassed of them and at that time really didn't understand why I had them.

Garfield Beach Towel

Toward the end of 5th grade, right before summer, we were all a little scared to go on to junior high school. Word on the street was that in P.E. we had to start taking showers. I think the main fear was that we were going to be naked and other kids would see us. Nobody wanted anyone else to see their ding-a-lings. This tripled as a problem for me because I didn't want anyone to see my jewels, belly, or huge knockers. I didn't care too much about my butt but certainly didn't want anyone to see the rest of my problems.

That summer, while everyone else was enjoying the break from school, I spent my time worrying about what I was going to do about this whole P.E. showering war I would be battling every day. At this point in my childhood, I still did not know that my heavy weight was because of eating so badly. I thought it was luck of the draw and I just got a horrible body while everyone else was blessed with normal bodies. I finally came up with the perfect plan. I was going to figure out how I could change in and out of my clothes and shower with a towel on. Unfortunately, regular shower towels didn't fit me but it just so happened that I had a giant Garfield the cat beach towel. It was bright blue, yellow and orange and I'm pretty sure it could've been used to wave airplanes in from miles away.

Every day, I practiced wrapping my upper and lower body with that towel while changing in and out of my clothes, just like a woman would. I practiced in the mirror, blindfolded, even in front of my mom so she could be impressed by what her son was able to accomplish on his own. I had it down pat. The only problem was... how was I going to casually carry a giant beach towel around with me all day at school with seven large textbooks as well?

The first day of P.E. was frightening. They handed out P.E. clothes to all of us (basically daisy duke shorts and tiny shirts – I think they mixed up the uniforms for guys and girls), talked about the upcoming year for P.E., and made us fill out forms to start our individual profiles for progress. At the end of class, we didn't have to shower. A huge weight lifted off my shoulders. Didn't seem so bad. But then I found out that not only would we be showering amongst ourselves but we would be sharing the locker room and showers with the 7th and 8th graders too. Sixty-plus guys? That's just too many guys sharing only six shower heads at the same time that were right next to each other. I had no idea how I was going to make it through the year in this situation.

The next class, we played a few games and again, no shower. Two weeks later, I hadn't slept much because the suspense was killing me and we still hadn't showered yet. I was beginning to think that maybe we'd skip it altogether but then the day came. At the end of class, the P.E. teacher yelled out, "let's hit the shower, boys!" I about fainted. There were only a few of us fat boys in the class. The others looked about the same as I felt inside: completely frightened. I think one kid was actually crying- which I was too, on the inside.

When we got into the locker room, all the regular-bodied guys stripped down like it was normal and they had done this before. *What the hell?* Maybe they practiced all summer, who knows? A few of the fat kids didn't seem to have a problem with it at all. One kid had tears in his eyes and started bawling because he didn't want to shower. The P.E. teacher was yelling at him, "Get your clothes off and get your ass in there! You have 30 seconds or you're getting detention." The kid ended up going through with it even though he was crying his eyes out.

I looked down at my 7-foot tall Garfield beach towel. It was ready for the magic show I was about to perform. I was embarrassed thinking about using it because nobody else was doing anything like this. I thought about that poor kid crying and how he did it even though his body was as bad, if not worse, than mine. By this time, guys were already coming back from the shower. The other P.E. teacher was standing at the exit of the showers handing towels out to everyone. The towels barely fit the skinny kids' waists: they were most definitely going to look like a washcloth on us sumo wrestlers. So, I faced my greatest fear and stripped down butt naked – boobs out, junk out, belly wobbling up and down; everything. I tried to walk fast, yet slow enough to not accentuate the moveable areas of my body, so I could hurry and get it over with. It was the scariest thing I ever had to do in public and even though it scared the hell out of me every single day after that, I faced one of life's scariest obstacles growing up as a kid.

Smart Puberty

I'll never forget how uncomfortable I always felt around girls when I was growing up. Occasionally, a girl would be mean or rude to me about my weight but it wasn't often, I think because I was always the nice and sweet boy in class. I couldn't ever talk to any of the girls that I liked because I was too self-conscious of everything about myself. I loved all of the girls but just the mere thought of saying hello to one of them made me almost go into convulsions. I was barely able to say hello to the ones I didn't have a crush on, especially in grade school.

It's always been a struggle for me to tell the girls I liked how I felt about them. However, I did try once with a girl when I was in fourth grade. I was head-over-heels completely in love this girl. My 10-year-old heart would beat a thousand miles per hour and be stuck in my neck at just the sight of her. I couldn't stop thinking about her and it only grew worse and worse each day. When I'd see her, my face would feel like it had needles poking out of it and my palms were sweaty. I had zero confidence in myself, so talking to her was completely out of the question. I finally found a way to *kind of* express my feelings to her. I'd get money from my mom and go buy little gifts from the stores at the plaza across the street from our apartments. Everyday, I'd secretly leave her little gifts with a small drawing along with the numbers *143*, which meant, "I love you." This went on daily for about a month until one day, my dumbass friend decided to tell her that they were all from me. I remember that scary moment. She turned around and looked at me shocked for a few seconds, made a weird face like she won toilet paper in a lottery, and that was the end of it. A few girls laughed and I was extremely embarrassed. I was so shy and that made it even worse for me. I never did anything like that again.

During puberty, my biggest weapon for being able to exchange a few words with girls was my perfect grades in school. I was always top of my class, so girls would come sit by me to get answers for homework they didn't do the night before. I think I purposely studied my ass off just for those few moments, which would last 2-3 minutes on average; 5 minutes on an awesome day. Those short interactions would make my entire day because I knew I had no other way of ever sharing time with any of them. I looked forward to it and always hoped we'd get tough homework just because I knew it would mean I might be able to *almost* talk to a girl.

Most of our conversations started with them asking if I did the homework, which they knew I did. I'd say, "yes" and bring it out for them. I tried to keep it in a trapper keeper, zipped up in my backpack just so I could spend the extra 15 seconds or so with them as I got my homework out for them to copy. I loved that they sat by me as they copied my homework. They always smelled so pretty and I'd occasionally feel their shoulder touch mine as they leaned over to read my work. Sometimes a light graze of their knee would touch mine. I started feeling less jealous of the non-fats in class and their gift of talking to girls anytime they felt like it because, by my book, I was getting some play too… sort of. I was happy: I felt there was hope for me to, one day, break away from being this super shy, sweet chubby boy who was afraid of so many things because of the way that he saw himself in the mirror. Worse case scenario, at least I was smart and maybe I could tutor girls the rest of my school years.

A Confident "Big Daddy" in Mexico

Big Daddy was an awful name given to me by my baseball coach in 8th grade. One of my greatest gifts growing up was my natural talent for all sports. I was overweight, yes, but I was extremely athletic. I was a fat athlete, or fathlete, if you will. I believe that because I was so athletically gifted growing up, I never really had any bullies. Of course, I had the verbal, joking bullies who made fun of me about my weight but it often times lead to a fun game of me throwing them down or hurling a ball eighty miles per hour at them. Sports really helped me with confidence in certain areas of my childhood and teen years. My favorite sports to play, which I was exceptional at, were baseball and basketball. They gave me a sense of belonging and who knows how fat I would've gotten had I not been so active growing up.

Each season, two players from each team were chosen to be part of the All-Stars baseball team and I was always one of the guys picked to play. I think my quiet nature, yet need to be noticed in the spotlight, came from my being the best pitcher in the league. The whole game, everyone had to watch me and as long as I was doing great, being fat didn't really matter. And I never had to say anything. I was a special player because not only was I the fastest pitcher with the most strikeouts, I was also the hardest hitter most of the years I played and I never got struck out. Baseball was my strength and I had great passion for it in my younger years.

One of my favorite memories was the time our team got to play the Mexican All-Star team in the Babe Ruth League, 14-year-old division. Coach told us that we would be going down to play on their field in Somerton, which made no sense to any of us. In Yuma, our biggest highlight playing baseball was that we got to use the professional field that the San Diego Padres used for Spring Training games. Why wouldn't they just come up and play on a real professional field we had access to? The name *Padres* is actually Spanish and they were the Mexican team so it seemed appropriate for them to want to come play there.

Our coach told us that we had to go play on their field. We were the best team in Arizona and had never lost but he told us that when we got down there to, "just have fun and do our best." Honestly, we had no idea what he meant or why he said that until we got down there. First, it was 110 degrees and in the middle of nowhere. The field had no fences, bases that were shred to pieces, no benches for the parents to sit on, holes all over the ground. Second base was a small bush (no joke) and there was a tree in left-center field. What the hell was this place? No dugout or fenced-in area for the players, just a splintery bench that about 6 kids could sit on. There was nothing to regulation about this place. The players all looked different ages. One guy had a full beard and mustache and looked like he was about 30 years old. I'm not positive but I think he was drinking a beer and had his wife and baby there cheering him on.

We quickly found out why our coach had told us to just

go and have fun. The umpires there were calling everything in favor of their team and everything against ours. They got all of their runs in by umpires calling balk on our team. *(Balk is when there are runners on base and the pitcher pretends to start pitching or shifts their shoulders when in position to pitch to trick the runners on base to try and pick them off for an out).* When they called balk on us, each runner got to advance a base – so on third base, a balk would score a run for them. Without getting too detailed in the game and the calls made, let's just say they were cheating. In All-Stars, its double elimination and their team would be out if they lost one more game. We were undefeated, so we could afford a loss and still be in it.

Just like a great baseball movie, we were in the bottom of the 9th inning, tie game, bases loaded, two outs, and a full count on the batter. I hadn't pitched at all that game. I guess the coach thought we were going to lose anyways and to save the arm for the next game or something. He decided to put me in to pitch. It came down to one pitch to either save the game or lose the game.

Their umpires didn't allow me to have any warm-up pitches. You're supposed to get 8 warm-up pitches before you pitch. I remember their coach, their parents, and the team telling the kid not to swing. The umpire was sure to call balk on me and walk the winning run in. It was in the bag for them. But, every kid batting in this situation has a dream of hitting a grand slam or at least get a hit to bring in the winning score. The batter was a small kid and the bat probably weighed as much as him. I knew as long as I threw it over the plate and just fast enough he'd go for it. I knew he wouldn't be able to keep up with bat speed, especially under the heat from *Big Daddy*. The biggest wave of disappointment flowed from everyone when I struck him out. Even the umps were pissed. We won that game and kept our perfect record.

Besides still being a lover of sports, I love that I was blessed with that talent as a kid growing up with poor self-esteem in my appearance. I had a taste of success in something that was physical and also developed what I believe to be a healthy competitiveness with both others and for myself.

Mom – The Natural Sweetener

In my career as a comedian, as well as a fitness instructor and trainer, I've had the pleasure of meeting many wonderful people from all over the world. My single most favorite person of all time was my mom. God rest her soul. She has been my best friend and always my biggest fan, even in the short time I've had with her in this life.

My favorite characteristic about her was her genuine kindness for every single person she'd ever been in contact with. I've had many sweet people in my life but none as much as her. She lived for her family and there were no boundaries to what she would do for our happiness. She was the perfect mom for me especially with the poor outlook I had about myself growing up. She gave me endless love, which I only ever felt from her alone, and nobody else, when I was growing up. She was overly perfect with her love toward me and never, ever stopped, even after she passed away – I can still feel it every day.

I bring up my mom because I feel that she was flawless in doing everything in her heart to make me feel good about myself. In my younger years, I heard a lot of terrible and painful insults, even from myself about myself, and she helped to keep balance in my own self-perception and my worth.

In junior high and high school, I had a very awkward appearance most of the time. I tried to hide my fat by wearing baggy clothing and long sleeve flannels, even in the 110º Arizona heat. I would rather feel miserable than look fat, even though I really wasn't hiding much from the world. I hated how I looked every moment of every day.

Even though my body looked how it did, my mom would always tell me how beautiful I was. I think she overshot quite a bit on occasion but that's okay, mothers tend to do that with their own kids. I would be getting ready to go to a school dance where I knew I stood no chance of dancing with any of the girls

I liked. I had on my Z Cavaricci clothes, tucked in shirt with a big belly and nice perky cone-like boobs sticking out. I was staring at myself in the mirror with disgust and my mom was standing behind me gloating about how handsome I looked: "Oh sweetheart! Look at you. You are going to break every girls' heart." I know what she was trying to do but that was a bit much. I'm not sure if she had poor eyesight or just really wanted me to believe in myself. She's standing there telling me I'm about to break hearts and I'm thinking of why the hell I look so awful. That was my attitude then and I probably was a product of my own bad energy. I never got to dance with any of the girls I had a crush on but that was ok. My mom told me it was because I was so handsome I made them nervous but I know the real reason – they weren't into Z Cavaricci...or big boys.

My mom really saved my self-outlook, even though I always struggled with my own image and hated looking at myself in a mirror. As of now, I have no kids but can only imagine how my mom felt when she was raising me. I was happy in some areas but completely sad in others. In the 3rd grade, not too long after my visit with my dad, I remember a time that I can't ever imagine a parent experiencing with their child. Unfortunately, I remember it and I wish I didn't. We were pulling into our apartment complex on our way home when I suddenly broke out in tears. I was crying hard and my mom had no idea what was going on. When she asked me what was wrong, I told her that I wanted to die, that I hated myself and I just didn't want to live anymore. I remember seeing her cry and hold me. Maybe she knew what was going on, maybe she didn't. All I know is that she made it her passion to always make me feel loved, wanted, and worthy.

Humor is a Powerful Weapon

Humor has always been one of my greatest characteristics. It helped me through many times growing up, from kids teasing me and gaining street cred to getting a girlfriend and eventually making a career for myself.

Although I'm known to be a great clean act in comedy for numerous types of events, it wasn't always the case. I wasn't always completely vulgar but I did say anything that would get a laugh out of friends and of course, girls. In high school, I was still the shy, quiet type but was also known for having a fun sense of humor. I remember some good friends who I could make laugh until the point of blacking out. Those were some of the best times of my life.

Quick wit was born in me from having to react to other kids insults growing up. As long as you had the funnier cut-down, it didn't matter what they said about you. It was more about who had the better and funniest comeback.

One particular friend shared many of the same characteristics as I did, except he wasn't fat – he was the opposite, very little. We had so many funny times and I think it was those days that helped me find my voice in this world. We laughed just about every single day to the point where we couldn't breathe. A lot of pie-in-our-face type of joking but we occasionally went after someone if the opportunity was available. We once had an art class together in high school because we were both super into drawing. One kid we sort of disliked, even though he was *kind of* our friend, used to draw superman type drawings and ninja drawings. That's all he ever drew. He was tall and had a loud, goofy and breathy type voice and we were excellent at impersonating his voice. One day, for whatever reason, we decided to take his drawings and add penises to as many of them as we could to enhance the drawing. We took his superman flying drawing and added a giant dong and balls with hair in his hand like he was flying away with it. We drew wiener nunchuks in the ninja's hand like he was swinging them. Some characters we made into a human unicorn with a big schlong coming out of his forehead. We must've marked up at least 20 of his drawings, doing 2 or 3 each day for about a week. Really childish stuff, really, but it was so funny to us. The first time he opened his folder up at his locker in the class, you could hear him, "Aw man, what the hell?" But then he stared at the drawings like he enjoyed it. Every day it was, "Aw man, what the hell?" but then he'd stand there and stare for a few minutes, smiling. The funniest part was when the teacher found them. She stared at the drawings for a long time, like she enjoyed them as well. We were the class clowns and troublemakers in the class and I'm pretty sure she knew we were responsible.

Humor has given me strength to do things I've never had the courage to. Not only have I gone from a shy and quiet boy into standing in front of audiences of hundreds to thousands of people, I have been able to communicate effectively in situations that I've felt uncomfortable in. The first girl I ever felt I couldn't live without was won over by my humor and personality. Even though I looked like I was a punchline, she was in love with the person my humor has helped me to become.

Joking around and laughing helped me deal with much of the stress I had growing up. I often times watched standup comedy on television and HBO because I liked how it made me feel. As I matured, I felt my humor was best when I kept it universal and not singling one person out for the sake of laughter. From a health standpoint, I believe we need to laugh every day. We can balance out problems by seeing the comedy in it. One definition I always liked about the word was: *comedy is pain plus time.* This means that in time, we should let go of the hardship and find joy in it. Don't dwell on our problems and grow from them by beating them and moving on. Humor, to me, is an essential part of our health and wellbeing. There are many physical and chemical benefits to laughing but I see it as a sign of good attitude, kindness, creativeness, and purposely choosing to see the good in situations.

Shock the World

After my crazy night of madness at 18, when I could've ended such a beautiful life-to-be, I decided that I was going to lose weight and be different. I was tired of being who I was and looking how I looked. I wanted to be good looking. I wanted to be hot. I wanted to be wanted by the opposite sex.

Upon shaving my head and discovering the Bruce Lee book that would change my life, I joined the gym. I used the book as my bible and applied everything in it to my life. The only thing that I did differently from the book was that I did more. I worked out as much as I could physically endure and ultimately became this exercise and diet maniac. For motivation to remind me each day to be strong, I had Bruce Lee pictures up all around my broken up room, covering the holes in the walls and doors. I also kept a very strict daily journal that I wrote in each time I worked out or ate. I'd write out the exact workout I did, the duration of it, how many sets/reps/weight it was, the time I did it, and so on. I weighed in each morning and at night, as well and logged it in my book.

One of my preferred cardio workouts was jump roping every day. I started only being able to do 1 minute and worked into a full 60-75-90 minute continuous without stop in a matter of a couple months. I did abdominal workouts for 90 minutes per day, including a 30-minute crunch regimen to warm up, and eventually developing a full 8-pack stomach with the strict diet I was on. I lifted weights every morning for 90 minutes. Of course, the book didn't list these as the recommended regimen but I did them anyways and explored my own abilities and likes. I wanted to find my limits and see what I was capable of doing. I also wanted to lose weight really, really badly!

At this point of 85 pounds lost, I hadn't seen or hung out with any friends the entire time. It was a shock waiting to happen. I finally decided to see everyone. Nobody recognized me, not a single person. Some laughed and some were shocked, and most couldn't look me in the eyes. This was exactly what I wanted. I was no longer the shy, fat guy. I was the fittest and most in shape of every single person I knew. No more double extra large shirts, my shirts were all mediums now. I had a new body and I never wanted to go back to the person I was before. I had worked very hard for it and was very proud of myself.

The key to this weight loss and life change was all inside of me. I wanted it so badly and so I did it. I had the help of a book that I sought out to start my journey but ultimately, it was me who did this transformation. I made a goal, started my planning, and did it. I did it alone too. I enjoy working out with others and having friends who share this area of my life with me but when it comes down to it, I am doing this for myself. It's a great thing to find people to do healthy things with but at the end of the day, fitness is a self-sport. Our friends aren't with us every workout or every meal and they don't know our every thought. We have to decide what we want out of this entire wellness industry and just go get it with full focus and intention. The decision is ours to make and we are in full control of what we choose to do or choose not to do.

It's an ongoing, endless, and amazing journey in which we will never stop learning. We always have something to strive for and limitless ways to better ourselves. I've had a lot of ups and downs in my life after the weight loss but exercise has never left my life. It is one of my *power-ups* and it can always make me feel better no matter what is going on in my life. It's something I look forward to every day and something I wish to always share with the world. I'm happy that I discovered it early enough in life that it's become a fixture that will always be present and a part of me. In the beginning, it was about looking good and impressing others. Whether or not that's a factor to me now, I definitely know that it's a part of me because I love myself and want to be my best in everything I have and do.

Group
Challenge

Each class, we do a group challenge. It's a collaboration of hard work, expression, strengths, weaknesses, and our motivation together as a group. In this section of the book, we will hear some wonderful short stories from people who wanted to share with the world. They are all different types of people who decided to participate for the purpose of this book – to connect with people who want to change and put exercise into their lives.

The introductions to each story was written by me. Each participant gave me a little information about them and I also added in some of my own descriptions.

Forward
By Brian Barabe

"The boot camp class begins in eleven minutes and the tall, tanned, shaven-headed instructor is laying out black rubber exercise mats at points around the room. A handful of class participants help position mats, plastic steps, and dumbbells. A few more participants come in. At five minutes before class it looks like it'll be a small group, only twelve or thirteen, this day. At one minute before class there are thirty-four people and more are coming through the door.

The instructor begins by explaining the exercises to be done at each station, making teasing quips as he speaks. He announces a young woman's thirty-fifth birthday and says she has set the group challenge for the day: thirty-five pushups in thirty-five seconds, another quip. Finished with the explanation, he starts at the first station and has the class repeat what the exercises will be. Energetic music plays though the speakers overhead. This is how Robby Wagner's class begins.

Throughout the hour Robby encourages individuals and small groups. His voice rings with energy and positivity. He keeps us posted as to when an exercise minute is about to end and the next one to begin. He watches individuals and models the exercise if they are doing the exercise wrong.

At both warm-up and cool-down time, he leads us through some slow stretches with pleasant music. During cool-down he reminds us of when and where his other classes are held. He also sends his weekly schedule out via Facebook, which has enabled him to keep a steady and growing following.

After class, Robby generously shares exercise ideas, advice, and more encouragement. He also shares what he has read about diet. And even after class he is still full of laughter and jokes. He's a total fitness instructor. It's a wonder to be part of something so dynamic that brings so many different personalities, ages, backgrounds and ethnicities together."

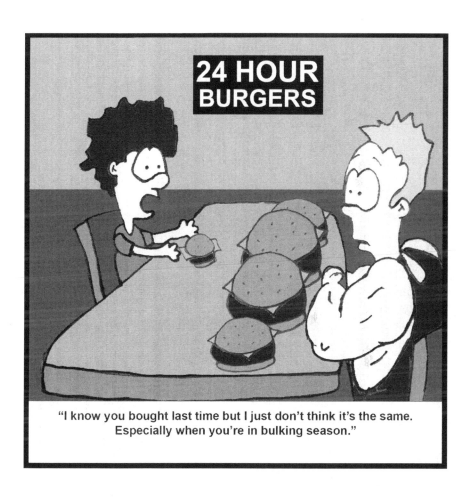

"I love the person I've become, because I fought to become her."
- Kaci Diane

KRISTA

This person I'm introducing is not just my friend but someone that makes me always want to be better in my own life. Her name is Krista and she's a 34 year-old German/Italian woman from New Jersey who is now living in Gilbert, Arizona. If you ever ask her what her favorite hobbies are you would feel the need to start out by saying, "Besides exercising...". Day in and day out, you'd think going to the gym would just become a habit of "just going" but you can count on her not failing to get the most out of her visit every single time. I've noticed that there are some people who attend class who have no idea that they have the gift to motivate others to be the best they can be – they just do it by their presence and energy. Krista definitely is this person. I could tell you many of her favorite things, such as, her favorite exercise is various types of planks and her favorite cheat food is steak, but I think her story will let you know the kind of person she really is.

I was pleased to learn about the mountains she's moved in her life and I think it'll always be something that reminds me of my own personal strength. I don't have a single observation about her but, instead, many that are positive. However, one word I associate with her is "strong" because it fits her well in every aspect I see and know about her. I'm really proud to have her be a part of this book, a part of my own journey in fitness, and without a doubt, a dear friend. Thank you for sharing such a wonderful story with the world, I know many will take much from this and there are people out there who need to see how amazing and powerful exercise can be.

Without further adieu, here's Krista's story:

I am a total Libra when it comes to my journey with fitness. I went from one extreme to the other, finally now finding a place where there is balance.

As a kid, I loathed sports and exercise of any kind. I would much rather be buried in a book than anywhere near a gym. I was the quintessential short, fat girl that would be the last picked for everything. When I went to college, I found a love of drinking and partying that masked my inner sadness for many years. That continued even after I got my first job teaching elementary school. Still no exercise, but lots of binge drinking, binge smoking and binge eating. The only time I was happy was when I was with my students. After school, I would lock myself in my apartment and eat and eat and eat.

Basically, I was eating myself to an early grave. I was almost 300 pounds at only 4 foot 10 inches tall. I didn't care, honestly.

But one day, someone else cared. A co-worker of mine invited me to a bootcamp class that her husband ran. I went, and I failed miserably. I couldn't even walk on a treadmill without my knees buckling. I was a mess, but I went back. I figured, might as well. At least someone cares about my physical well-being when I sure don't.

Fast forward a few years. By sheer determination, some horrific diets, and more exercise than was healthy (4-5 hours a day), I had lost over 150 pounds. At my lowest, I was 93 pounds, and honestly, anorexic. I had transferred all of my bad habits into over-exercise and starvation. And I was still miserable. However, at least now I loved working out and meeting fit friends and jumping. I never ever in my life could jump, and now I was like a little bunny. But the second I left the gym, I would feel sad. The depression came to the point where I just couldn't handle my life anymore. I was not happy fat and I was not happy skinny. I decided to end my life.

I don't know if it was a higher power or what, but I survived my suicide attempt. I didn't want to, but there I was. I failed at dying, so I might as well try living again. After spending a few days at the "mental spa," I had help learning how to eat normally and sometimes take a break from working out. It released a lot of monsters, and when I returned to the gym, I found myself enjoying it so much more.

Exercise has been part of me ever since. It is my emotional release and when I can most be myself. Finding my passion in boxing and bootcamps has been more powerful than therapy for me, and I usually workout twice a day. I now can love my body for its short-comings (pun intended) and strengths. I love challenging myself and seeing my instructors smile when I am doing something well. When I am in bootcamp, which is usually twice a week, I feel surrounded with people who don't judge but share a common goal of loving ourselves. Every single person in those classes has overcome personal demons. Bootcamp is for us to be safe, laugh and push ourselves to finish class sweating and smiling. There is nothing else like it. Jump overs, one regular station which uses steps, are still my biggest challenge. I really love doing planks of all variety, and several of my fitness friends often remark that I seem to have endless endurance.

I love telling people to not be scared or intimidated by a bootcamp class because, really, even if they think they failed miserably, it's a victory just to participate, and an even greater victory to come back.

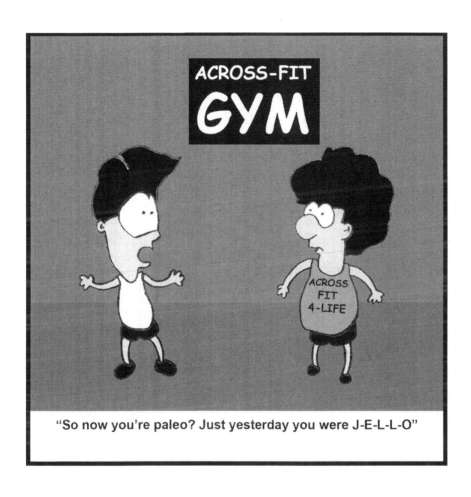

"The way you think, the way you behave, the way you eat, can influence your life by 30 to 50 years."

- Deepak Chopra

BERNICE

I don't even know where to start when introducing one my favorite people in the world. It's an understatement to say this woman makes my soul smile ear-to-ear. Bernice is a 74 year-old woman from Winnemucca, Nevada that is married with one daughter and two granddaughters. For her birthday this year, the class did 74 Spiderman push-ups as a challenge because it is her favorite exercise. I typically see her twice a week for bootcamp and once for cycling. Like many others, I look up to this woman who is so strong and so sweet. While a few will say they hope to be in the shape she's in when they're her age, most will tell you they wish they were in her shape now. The last couple years have been amazing to get to know this extraordinary woman. She loves to travel with her husband and/or friends and she has a heart for animals and volunteering. The days I see Bernice are days that I look forward to teaching. There's never a time I don't get greeted with a hug that is filled with so much love and caring that my own stresses cease to exist anymore. As mentioned before, she is one of my favorite people in the world and I love her very much!

Without further adieu, here's Bernice's story:

The reason I started exercising 40 years ago was not to lose weight, but to manage stress. At the time I was just 30 years old and in a highly dysfunctional marriage. I decided to run off the stress. I was employed at ASU in the athletic department. So during my lunch hour I would go to the track and field arena and run around the track. At first, I could only run once around the track, which was a huge accomplishment for me at that time. But, as I kept running, I was able to increase my mileage which built up my confidence. Then, I began exploring other types of exercise. Aerobics had become popular, so I would find free classes. I really enjoyed the challenge and also meeting others who liked to exercise. We had a common ground and to this day I still have friendships from that season of my life.

I became an exercise enthusiast immediately because I saw the changes in me physically and mentally. Eventually, I joined a gym and began lifting weights 3-4 times a week. Exercising was an outlet for me that I have not stopped. By building up my confidence and gaining support from my circle of friends, I was able to walk away from my dysfunctional marriage and happily have never looked back. I also became the first member of my family to earn a BA in organizational communications and a minor in marketing during that hard season of my life.

I have been blessed with good health and have not had any medical conditions to prohibit me from exercising. I grew up on a huge cattle ranch: worked hard, ate organic food-which was not called organic at the time, did not have sodas to drink or candy to eat. Therefore, I believe through that healthy lifestyle I now, at this age of 73, still have good health.

I started taking Robby's bootcamp about 2 years ago after a friend invited me several times. I have to say, there were many exercises that I enjoyed and had never done before, but BURPEES was one that I had never even heard of. At first, they were incredibly hard. And honestly, they are still hard, but I can do them for the full time asked of me. I don't know if I actually excel in class, but do enjoy the challenge. One of my favorite stations is wall kicks. That movement has really tightened up my obliques and I like the change in my waist line. One of my favorite things about bootcamp has been getting to know Robby, the most awesome bootcamp instructor ever. Robby is always positive, loves to see the class have fun, but yet will challenge us. He really works hard and I will always be thankful for him. We have grown into close friends. His class is a fantastic workout for me and I feel so accomplished when it's over.

I love the fact that I have met so many wonderful classmates; also how much my body has slimmed down. I love spin classes, still run, swim, lift weights and use other machines in the gym. Now that I am retired, I work out 5-7 days a week. One of the reasons I work out so much is because

I love going to bootcamp as often as I can. My level of fitness may be considered above average because I have been exercising for the past 40 years. I am older than most people in classes at the gym, but I feel as strong or stronger than most. My strength is that I never give up and love to meet new challenges. My weakness is that I expect more of myself. I am a perfectionist, so if I can't do everything at every station sometimes I can be really hard on myself. But the class community has helped me in this area. I get so much support from everyone and so many compliments throughout class that I have begun to be more at peace with myself and my progress.

Taking boot camp, has affected all areas of my being. I now push myself harder when doing other exercises. Feeling good about myself has helped me in my relationships with my family, new marriage, etc. Although, I have always watched what I ate, I am now more aware of my meals-make sure I get the right amount of protein, water, and vegetables. Nutrition is about health, not just looks.

In my opinion, when you feel good about yourself and have a positive attitude it really affects all aspects of your life and that is why I keep exercising. I enjoy the social aspect and have amazing friendships. I feel if I can bring joy into another person's life by just being myself, I have been blessed.

I feel that no matter what age you are or what your situation, you should always take care of yourself because if you do not, it is almost impossible to take care of others. If you love yourself, you will be able to give love. Exercise is something that you can do for yourself and by doing so, will reap great benefits. Never be intimidated by anyone. We all are not alike and each one of us will excel at something- just need to find out what. Always, always, follow your passion for life.

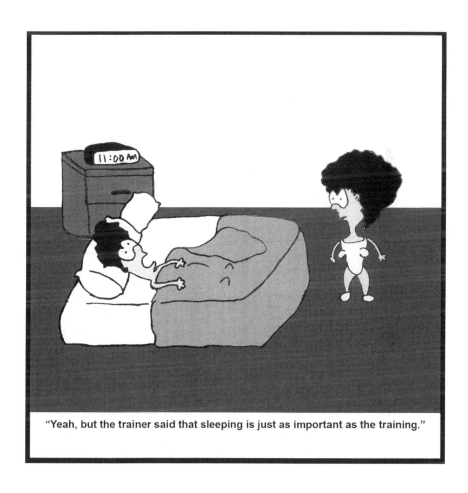

"Without health life is not life; it is only a state of languor and suffering - an image of death."

- *Buddha*

DERRICK

There's a lot to say about this next friend of mine. His name is Derrick and he's a married, 43-year-old tough guy from Oklahoma with a 22-year-old daughter. When I say tough, I don't mean just in class while training, I mean he could probably take on a dozen or so guys at once without flinching. I once saw him punch the heavy bag in class and 5 guys in the other room fell down from the aftershock of the hit. Some of his hobbies include: fitness, Jeeping, tactical firearms training (and filming them), chocolate stout beer and hiking. Derrick works as an Indoor Environment Quality Consultant, a.k.a. Industrial Hygienist. All his friends insist on meeting him out somewhere when they hang out so they don't get written up for having a messy home if he visits. Anyone who works out alongside him in class knows that he's the real deal and doesn't just look the part. He's always adding more to the workout that is laid out, mixing in a lot of creative modifications and often times, doubling the intensity of the exercises. He came to an outdoor bootcamp I held on Memorial Day and was dressed in army gear with an additional 40-50 lbs of weight on his back. He wore it, completing the entire bootcamp in insane Arizona heat. Derrick is definitely the friend you want behind you if something goes down and more importantly, he's the friend you want in your life, simply because he's just an amazing, well-rounded person who will probably do just about anything to help you out and is just happy for your friendship in return.

Without further adieu, here's Derrick's story:

There are a lot of miles on this 43-year old body of mine. It has propelled me into many fantastic adventures: surfing the Hawaiian North Shores, mountain biking in Colorado, wrestling in the Oklahoma State Championship, hiking the mountains of Philmont Boy Scout Ranch, kayaking the jungles of Costa Rica, dynamic room clearing with an armed assault team, motorcycling from Los Angeles, CA to Key West, FL and back, snowboarding, scuba Diving, water Skiing and many, many more. Aside from an unquenchable sense of adventure, what made all these escapades possible? Strength, endurance and confidence.

As an Eagle Scout I am committed per the Scout oath to keep myself physically strong, mentally awake and morally straight. I also have a hero complex. I am willing to run into the fray to save the lives of my family, friends and fellow citizens. But willingness is not the same as ability. Being as fit as possible ensures I can assist myself and others to my maximum capacity.

I used to be the quintessential 97-pound weakling. I was smart and small, therefore picked on a fair amount. But, I knew with consistent hard work, I could overcome the physical limitations and overwhelm the competition, who were coasting on their laurels. But the strength I eventually gained could not stop me from a wicked crash on my mountain bike a few years ago. It literally destroyed my shoulder. It took major surgery with wires and titanium, all the king's horses and all the king's men to put it back together again.

After three months of torture in a rigid sling, I could not raise my atrophied arm over my head. Three more months of rehab, I still couldn't perform one push up. With my strength, endurance and confidence smashed against the rocks, I needed an exercise option that would allow recovery from this historic fitness low back to a state of tuned health. LA Fitness Group Fitness Classes and Robby Wagner's Boot Camp Class filled the bill as the exercise option I needed. Now, I can once again drop and give you 80 pushups. Strength, endurance and confidence restored. I have been working out in Robby's bootcamps for about three years now. The classes provide me with a variety of benefits. I get to...

a.   Keep my aging body tuned to its capacity.

b.   Forget about the worries of the day.

c.   Do burpees next to my 65-year old mother, who attends the classes too.

d.   Surround myself with folks who are committed to a healthy lifestyle.

e.　　See men and women from ages 18 to 80 standing shoulder to shoulder giving their all to meet the instructor's challenges of the day.

f.　　Watch the progress of participants, who can only do 5 pushups on their knees their first day of class, crank out full pushups for a solid minute after only a few months of hard work.

g.　　Exercise in a nonthreatening, non-competitive environment with smiling sweaty faces all around.

I stay committed to fitness for a number of reasons: I want to be able to walk on the beach with my wife when I am 75. I want to be able to tie my shoes when I am 85. And, when my time comes, I want to be able to wrestle the Grim Reaper to the ground and give him a noogie before he takes me to forever more.

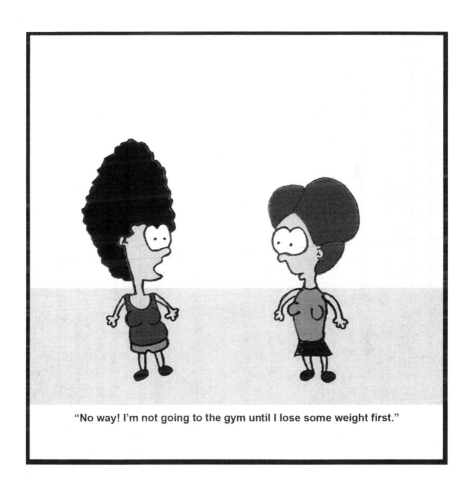

"No way! I'm not going to the gym until I lose some weight first."

"I'm so unfamiliar with the gym, I call it James."
- Ellen Degeneres

STEPHANIE

Whether it's a gift or not, there are some people that make you happy just by seeing their smiling face. This next person is one of those people in my life who makes things better just by being in the same room with me. Her name is Stephanie and she is just an amazing person, mother and friend to many. She's a 65 year-young Italian female from Brooklyn who decided to make Tempe, Arizona her home. She's married and has two sons that get their strength from their mom. Fun fact, one of those sons happens to be the story right before this one...Derrick the tough guy. She also has 3 grandkids that she's very proud of. One thing I noticed about Stephanie is her endurance in bootcamp, she claims it's because she's Italian and tomato sauce runs in her blood. I know that she loves photography and likes to take pictures of her other hobbies, which include food, exercise, and travel. It's unknown if she likes astronomy or not but she does love Milky Way bars. I asked her what her favorite classes were and she said bootcamp and an extreme distant second place, Zumba.

Without further adieu, here's Stephanie's story:

I started running to enjoy the outdoors after work. I was surprised how quickly my endurance built and I could run further as the days went on. I benefited from the famed "runner's high" and felt good overall. I wasn't overweight or in poor shape when I started, however, my body reacted by growing stronger and more toned, which was a great benefit.

Then, after a car wreck that caused damage to my neck, part of my therapy included exercises to strengthen my neck and upper body. Once I recovered, I began going to a gym for the first time. I worked out on the floor with machines and took classes, both Zumba and bootcamp. I enjoyed the benefit of being part of a group with the same goals as myself. I started working out 3-4 times a week and have kept that schedule. Some weeks I add 1 or 2 workouts in my home with DVDs I enjoy.

In the beginning, bootcamp was challenging yet enjoyable at the same time. Pushups were a challenge and I began with only a few on my knees. Now I am proud to say my pushups are on my toes and I can usually complete the class challenges. Even before joining the gym I would say my level of fitness was pretty good, but I have seen solid measurable growth and results. This is why I am hooked. Sit-ups are still a weakness, but, have no doubt, I am working on that.

Robby keeps the class enjoyable with his wit and encouragement. First he greets us with a friendly smile and tells funny stories while we warm up. Throughout the class, he checks our form for proper execution and safety. He continually encourages individuals as he walks around the room. His fun and caring personality really make the class a stand out. Taking bootcamp with my son is an extra perk.

Another benefit of bootcamp is that I've learned about eating more protein to build muscle and increase my stamina. With the strength I've gained I'm able to add more weight to my workouts as well. My stress factory has gotten smaller since I started working out, which rolls over into bettering my personal and work life. I am most proud of myself for all the effort I put forth in my workouts. Exercise is a great stress relief for me and I feel incredible after a hard workout.

We have been given one body and it is our responsibility to respect and care for it. Let those words sink in and then move forward toward a healthy and happy life. Robby's goal as an instructor is to make sure you succeed with your own goals. Meeting your goals and then blowing past them is an amazing feeling. Working out under an instructor who fosters a fun group atmosphere with great music that keeps you moving is one hour worth living through. Only one WARNING: bootcamp is addictive.

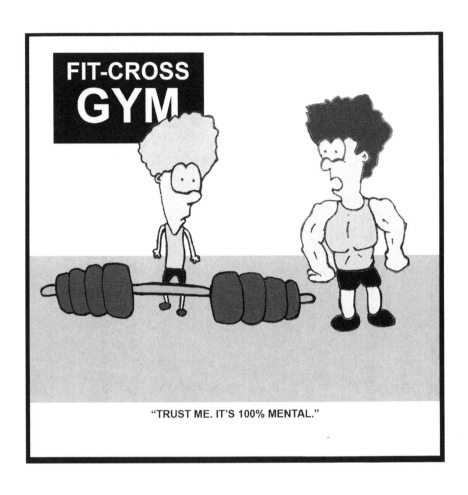

"Its bizarre that the produce manager is more important to my children's health than the pediatrician."

- Meryl Streep

SARAH

This next person is nothing less than a powerhouse athlete and sweetheart of a girl who I've had the pleasure of becoming friends with in her short time living in Arizona. Her name is Sarah and she is a 25 year-old Costa Rican from Houston, Texas that is a soon-to-be Doctor of Physical Therapy. She enjoys fixing people, Acro Yoga, triathlons, cycling, and doing handstands. Her favorite food is sushi and her favorite cheat food is sushi. I think it's safe to say she takes more cheat days than most athletes you see. She also said she's "so single" and her favorite exercises are deadlifts, manmakers, and lifting people – I'm not sure if those two things are a cause-and-effect situation but it would make for great conversation over a plate of sushi. That, or the fact that she's already completed a full Ironman. Whether or not she knows it, Sarah has an amazing energy that motivates anyone that is working out near her. She has a positive competitiveness about her that seems to help others push themselves harder than they normally would. She's a great person to train with because if you pass out, she'll dead lift you, lift you up, and almost always find a way to manmake you. If not, she'll roll you up like sushi and put you in a safe place until you recover.
Without further adieu, here's Sarah's story:

Life often brings us full circle. Having struggled before with finding a healthy relationship with my body, I decided to become an ACSM certified personal trainer. It's funny how once you become a personal trainer; you think things will be easier. The truth is, I'll never shy away from a workout-- but sometimes the couch is really comfortable and cookies definitely still taste good. It's for reasons like this that I've learned the power of community and encouragement to facilitate growth.

Before I started bootcamp I was definitely in good shape, but not feeling as great as I could have. I have always been strong for a girl, but I was struggling with my self-image at the time. I was visiting Arizona for the summer for a physical therapy rotation and a friend invited me to come to bootcamp with her. The burpees and squats were a challenge; I can tell when I haven't been doing them because it takes me a while to get back into it. I loved being a part of a group of people working out and being able to compete! Honestly, I look around in class and tell myself I want to be first. It's just that athlete in me coming out to play. This dynamic of bootcamp keeps the workouts fun and fresh.

Not only did I get stronger and fitter in bootcamp, but my mood and relationships benefited as well. It's hard for me to be vulnerable and I often keep my problems to myself. Bootcamp provided me a network of like-minded people that were strong and willing to hear my story. I met a ton of awesome people, and even though I am back in Texas now, we are still friends.

Since bootcamp, the journey has only continued. I have participated in various races, competitions, and events. However, my focus has shifted more from myself to other people. As I will graduate in May 2016 as a Doctor of Physical Therapy, I often think back to the strength that I have drawn from my friends to be able to overcome various obstacles. I hope I can continue to share my passion for fitness and general wellness in a way that my patients can feel it and continue to spread the empowerment throughout the nation and even the world.

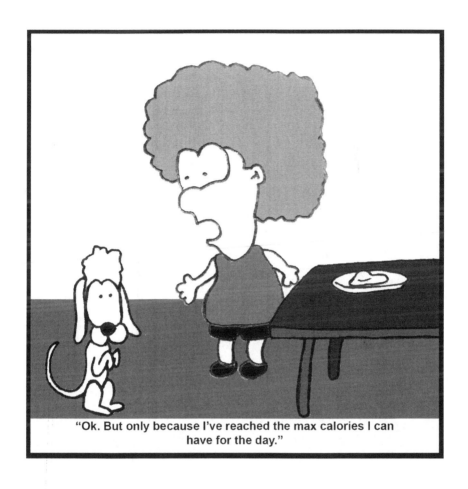

"Ok. But only because I've reached the max calories I can have for the day."

"Want to learn to eat a lot? Here it is: Eat a little. That way, you will be around long enough to eat a lot."

- Anthony Robbins

MUNA

I'm happy to have the pleasure to introduce to you my friend, Muna Ali. She's from a small town outside of Arizona called Somalia. She works at DES and recently won my bootcamp "strongest social worker from East Africa that is now living in Arizona and is 35 years old" contest. Aside being the same age as I am, I noticed that our hobbies seem to match up well too. She likes to cook and clean and I love to eat and not clean up after myself......ever. Word on the street is that she is an incredible chef. However, her favorite cheat food of choice is hamburgers. When I asked if she likes cheeseburgers, she shook her head no and slapped me in the face with an Angus patty...uncooked. And even though I'm vegetarian, I have to say that was probably the best tasting, uncooked burger I've ever been slapped with. She is a single mother of 4 kids, which basically means that no bootcamp in the world is as tough as this woman is. I'm very pleased that she enjoys class regularly and I'm even happier that she chose to share her story with everyone. Thank you for your friendship, I'm blessed to have you as my friend.
Without further adieu, here is Muna's story:

I haven't always exercised. After marriage, my move to the United States and having a baby, I wasn't happy with my weight. But I lacked motivation to workout. Being mistaken as my husband's mother when I was pregnant with our second child gave me that motivation. I was stunned when someone asked if I was his mother. Right then I said to myself, *I need to change my life.* Coming from a diabetic family also pushed me toward creating a healthier lifestyle.

Six years ago I joined a small women's gym, Curves, and went on the Slim Fast diet (not the best diet but at the time that's what everyone was doing). Getting into the workout mood was the hardest part of this new lifestyle for me. Curves was a good kick start to my fitness – I enjoyed lifting weights but was weak in cardio strength. It took me about a year to really get addicted to exercise, but once I did, I wanted more.

43

Eventually I moved over to LA Fitness, where I watched group classes through the glass dividers. The women in the bootcamp class seemed so strong. The exercises looked fun and challenging. I wondered if I would ever be strong enough to complete such a class. The challenge allured me. You don't even know you can do those types of movements until you try. I planned to go to class 5 times, and hung back, watching 5 times before I actually went inside. Five months ago I walked through the group fitness room and participated in my first bootcamp class. It was so hard! I loved it. Now I take two bootcamp classes a week. The more you do bootcamp, the more you discover yourself.

Before I joined bootcamp I worked out six days a week. Over time I lost most of my baby weight and got a lot stronger and more confident. Now, I only workout four or five days a week but have lost even more weight, and I am a lot stronger. For me, the bootcamp style of workout mixed with step classes and gym floor time is a really good way to get fit. Even putting in less time I have become so much stronger. Exercise has made me feel good about myself and increased my energy levels. Bootcamp has helped lower my stress level and boosted my energy even more. When social work gets draining I go to the gym to destress.

My favorite part about taking bootcamp is the motivation I get from our instructor, Robby. His motivation helps me challenge and push myself to do more than I ever could before. My favorite stations are the ones that focus on strength. I love pushing myself and seeing what new level I achieve.

No one would think I am older than my age now. My friends and even my kids are never surprised when I break out dancing to energetic music. Exercise is the best way to change your life. It boosts self-esteem, improves energy levels and makes you feel really good about yourself. I'm so glad that I made the time for fitness in my life. I enjoy all the positive people in class. And I know I am making my life better whenever I go. One quote I love is, "Life is what you make out of it. Try your best without competing with anyone but yourself." The woman who I left behind six years ago will never come back: I am too happy and confident now, too healthy, to ever quit exercising.

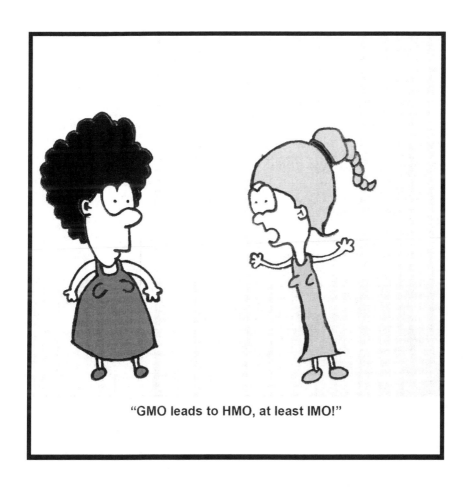

"GMO leads to HMO, at least IMO!"

"Strength does not come from winning. Your struggles develop your strengths. When you go through hardships and decide not to surrender, that is strength."

- Arnold Schwarzenegger

JIMMY

*What can I say about this next guy? He's one of the
kindest and most well rounded guys that I know. His name is
Jimmy and he's a single, 26 year-old Asian from Tempe, Arizona.
He has a love for fitness and sports and he's definitely a trained
athlete, as you would guess just by seeing him. One of his hobbies
is martial arts. I don't believe anyone in class would be surprised
to learn this after seeing his violent, fast kicks during our
workouts. It's an awesome thing to witness but also a thing to
watch out for if you're not paying attention. One time, just for
fun, he kicked one of the heavy bags off the chain and it landed in
the bathroom across the street at a Starbucks...while someone
was in there using it. Aside from sports and working out, Jimmy
enjoys jazz music, which actually seems to fit his easy going and
calm attitude perfectly. He loves a great Filet Mignon and when
he has cheat meals, he likes to have a burger from Rehab Burger
Therapy. I don't know what that place is but it sounds
dangerous. I'm very thankful for his friendship and couldn't be
any happier that he chose to be a part of this book.*

Without further adieu, here's Jimmy's story:

I started exercising when I was 18 because I wanted to
increase my stamina. I wanted to run longer and faster,
because I was an avid runner. Eventually, I also wanted to
build muscle mass. I wasn't fat, but I was what I call "skinny-
fat." I started with a few days a week at a gym. Not too long
after I started working out, I couldn't stop. Now, I am at 4-5
days a week. I work out on the gym floor, take kickboxing,
bootcamp, and occasionally run at night a few times a week. I
want to remain fit and maintain my health and build.

When I started taking bootcamp over a year ago, I was
looking for a cardio workout. I definitely received solid cardio
training, but also was surprised how difficult the leg exercises

were. Lunges, squats, and squat pulses were impossible for me. I gave out too quickly. I realized that I did not have strong leg strength. Taking this class has greatly improved my squats, and my finesse for martial arts. The kicking we do in class as well as other leg exercises empowers me in martial arts. Class has also helped improve my overall mood.

Exercise has definitely helped me become more confident and social. I really like how we're put in groups during bootcamp. I like the camaraderie of the team. Some people are nervous to come into class. I say, do it and don't be afraid. No one is looking at you. Everyone is working on themselves. If you fall, pick yourself up and dust yourself off to start again. Exercising is not something you should toil over, it's a lifestyle and a commitment. Once you get it running in full force, it is very difficult to stop because the benefits are so amazing.

Bootcamp has become one of my favorite workouts. I try not to miss any classes. Workouts that require use of the chest and triceps I tend to dominate. I also really enjoy the group challenges we do half way through class, and being able to see my progress in leg strength. Exercise has really helped my posture and made work days – which are sitting at a desk – easier on my back. Bench presses used to be most difficult for me on the gym floor but have now become my favorite exercise. Seeing such progress is addictive. Mentally I am also much healthier because of fitness.

I can't see myself ever moving away from this lifestyle. Now and then, I still lose my way, but I always get back. I love how I feel after a workout and the friends I have made in class who have the same health values as I do. I am known as the workout guy at work. I just can't help myself from inviting people to come to classes with me. Come! You won't regret it.

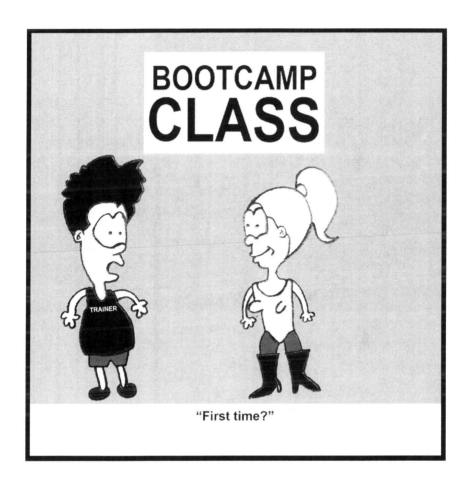

"Water is life, and clean water means health."
- Audrey Hepburn

TRACY

This next person I'm happy about introducing to you is Tracy. She is a beautiful 24 year-old grade school teacher from Tempe, Arizona. You don't find a lot of natives here in Arizona. You also don't find a lot of people that are in incredible shape like her either. I think at the rate she's going, you may just see a write up about her in a fitness magazine one day. I remember the first class she took of mine. She was in great shape already but now she seems like a super-athlete. Back when I would take endless bootcamp classes every day, I would've purposely been in whatever group she was at because I know she would've made me work harder. She definitely raises the bar and excels in every exercise that is laid out. I'm very happy to have a new friend who is as sweet as she is fit. I appreciate her for sharing her story to be a part of this book.

Without further adieu, here's Tracy's story:

Exercise became a huge part of my life in February of 2011. A week before Valentine's Day, my then-boyfriend of two years broke up with me. I knew I needed a goal to keep me healthy and happy. I signed up for a half marathon and had my first official training day on Valentine's Day. While that relationship did not work, my love for running has continued to this day. To date, I have run five half marathons and one full marathon. Without a doubt, I intend to run in more races.

Prior to joining bootcamp, I was definitely active. I would run several times a week and use weighted machines. My strength was obviously cardio and my weakness was weight lifting. Since joining boot camp, I have noticed an improvement in my strength. I used to struggle to do arm exercises such as push-ups. Attending weekly classes has helped to increase my endurance and push me past my previous limits. It has also had a positive effect on my emotional well-being. Working full-time and going to school can be overwhelming. Exercise provides a sense of balance and stress relief to my daily schedule.

My best piece of advice regarding fitness is to sign up for events (i.e. triathlons, 5ks, or any event of interest). It forces you to train and remain goal-oriented. Taking classes can also push you past limits you may not even know you had. You will never regret getting fit.

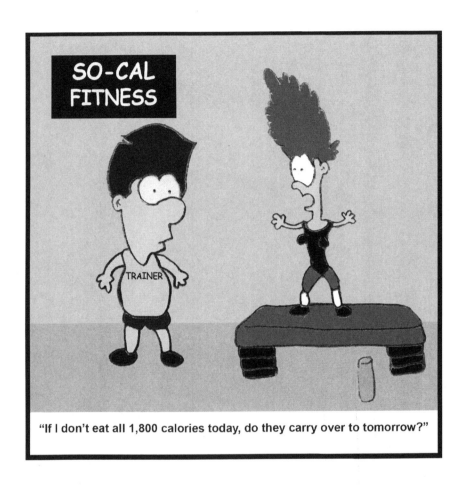

"If I don't eat all 1,800 calories today, do they carry over to tomorrow?"

"The difference between the impossible and the possible lies in a person's determination."

- Tommy Lasorda

RACHELLE

Let me introduce you to an extraordinary ex-deputy sheriff, Rachelle. She's a 49 year-old, African American woman from Milwaukee, Wisconsin – home of German sausage and beer! She has a "tough-as-nails" personality that matches up perfectly with bootcamp. Rumor has it that she once made Simon Cowell cry just by staring at him through the TV. Rachelle has one daughter and two grand children that don't take bootcamp class because they're only 7 and 8. She mentioned to me that she loves calamari as her cheat food of choice and I had to google what that was. My research shows that its squid and that made me realize she is definitely tougher than I thought she was! Her story is an inspiration and I know that it'll help many find their own strength within, just like her!

Without further adieu, here's Rachelle's story:

I was hit by a car in 2010 while walking on duty as a deputy sheriff in Wisconsin. The accident caused lasting injury to my knees. Then, in 2011 I was diagnosed with Breast Cancer, stage 3C, which left me with neuropathy in both my hands and feet along with lymphedema in my right arm. The lymphedema causes my arm to swell due to removal of 32 lymph nodes. During the diagnosis and treatment I lost myself and gained 75 pounds. So after relocating to AZ in 2013 I decided it was time to take back my life; I needed to get back to living.

I joined LA Fitness, got a personal trainer and began working out and changing my eating habits. It took me about six months to really love fitness. But once I began to see the changes my body made, I hated to miss any days at the gym. I went 6 days a week. Getting healthy became part of my lifestyle that I still continue to nurture and love.

When I first started bootcamp earlier this year I still couldn't do one push up. Now I can do sets of 10-12, 4 reps each, which shows me I am getting stronger. When I started class I considered myself beginner level. But I am quickly growing stronger! I have added to my 6 days a week an additional 4 evenings of bootcamps (so 4 of my 6 days are "2-a-days"). I also have incorporated walking 3 miles in the evenings that I don't take bootcamp. Now I can't imagine not giving myself this time to heal my body. The strength and exercise helps to balance out the pain that I have to live with.

My weakness at the beginning was being hard on myself because I couldn't run the laps or do the squats as I would have liked to. But I have the ability to push myself beyond my comfort zones without injuring myself. Each day I return to the gym I overcome a little of the physical challenges my accident and cancer have left behind. My new life has helped increase my energy. This is a priceless benefit, because my energy levels have been suppressed with all the meds I take to help keep cancer away. Fighting off these chemical side effects with exercise has enabled me to have a productive lifestyle. There are still days that I am unable to do many activities, due to the constant pain I am in. But overall, I will say exercise has drastically increased my quality of life.

I have met many people since joining the gym and taking bootcamp and Zumba classes. This has been helpful, because as I said, I am new to Chandler. My relationships have matured and are healthier. Growing stronger has also increased my confidence. My new life has helped me to make healthier food choices and drink only water. Also, my daily stressors have been greatly alleviated. My outlook on life is better than it was three years ago.

I would say to anyone who wants to take back their life: take it one day at a time and don't compare yourself to anyone else. You are a uniquely made individual and what works for one may not work for another. Also remember your age, because the older we are the harder it is for the weight to come off; but it will come off if you stay focused on the short and long term goals. Celebrate your small milestones. Never, ever give up.

NO REGRETS JUST RESULTS!!!!!

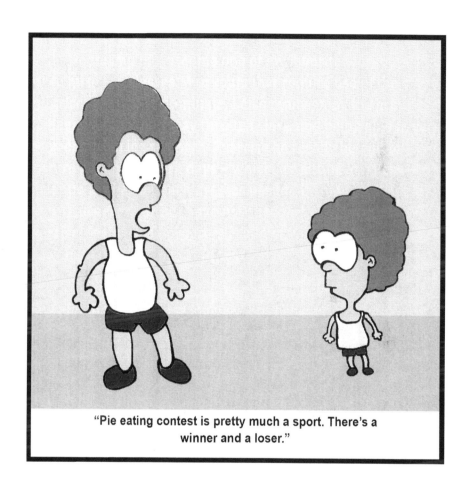

"Pie eating contest is pretty much a sport. There's a winner and a loser."

"Physical fitness is not only one of the most important keys to a healthy body, it is the basis of dynamic and creative intellectual activity."

- John F. Kennedy

Jimmy

I'm pleased to introduce my next friend to you. His name is Jimmy. Yes, there are two Jimmys in class and both are Asian. This particular Jimmy is the epitome of what the benefits of exercise can do for you. He's in his 50's but moves like he's in his teen years. I see him several times each week in class and always notice when he's not there. Whenever I put out a 'choose-your-own' cardio station, he always does burpees. I'm very happy that he chose to be a part of this book and to share his own story. Thank you for your friendship!
Without further adieu, here's Jimmy's story:

I have a lot of stress in work and personal life. A good workout tremendously helps me maintain a work/life balance. I am over 50 and have benefitted from Robby's dynamic, fun and sweaty bootcamp classes. I take at least one gym bootcamp and one park bootcamp a week.

About three or four years ago, I hurt my lower back while doing yard work. I received chiropractic treatment and went through about a dozen sessions of physical therapy. But the pain persisted. During the physical therapy sessions, I learned some key techniques to help heal my injury, such as strengthening all my back and core muscles. Joining Robby's boot camp more two years ago has been the most effective way to strengthen these muscles and it has worked really well. Planks, pushups, leg kicks, squats, mountain climbing, lunges, all help strengthen my core and back. Combined with my weekly hiking on mountains in the Valley of the Sun, my lower back is no longer a problem. I rarely notice the pain unless I sit at my desk for too long.

I initially tried Robby's classes after a recommendation from a friend. I was tentative because of my lower back and my busy schedule. Besides, how could I keep up in bootcamp with people who were much younger? The burpees plus many other exercises were hard. But, I pushed myself to keep it up. After a few weeks, my energy levels went up. I felt great after

57

each class. I am now sharper in business decision making. The best part is that my lower back pain is almost gone.

Every week, I look forward to Robby's classes. I shuffle my work meetings so that I don't miss classes. Robby rotates the stations and carefully chooses the music so that the classes are fun. With encouragements and laughs from fellow bootcampers, Robby's bootcamp is part of my weekly routine. I go to his classes three times a week and any time he adds one on. I brag about it and friends are jealous of my physical condition. When I hike across the Grand Canyon or climb up on Cactus to Cloud trail, many people in their 20's and 30's can't keep up with me. I am really happy with my pain-free, fit lifestyle.

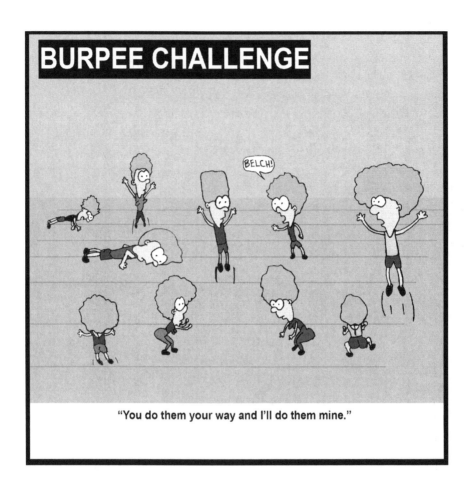

"To me, good health is more than just exercise and diet. It's really a point of view and a mental attitude you have about yourself."

- Albert Schweitzer

LAURENCE

I'm very honored to introduce this next woman to you. She is a very dear friend and an amazing person with a great story. Her name is Laurence and she is a 40 year-old married woman who works as a teen volunteer coordinator for Hospice of the Valley. Although born in Tempe, Arizona, she actually grew up in Lyon, France and is able to speak, hear, think and swear in several languages. She loves chocolate and is pitching the idea to Hershey's to come out with a new line: Hershey's Chocolate French Kiss. When she's not watching TV shows or reading magazines, she enjoys going to happy hour with friends and not enemies. I had the pleasure to learn quite a bit about this incredible woman this year as she faced some tremendous obstacles. I used to see her sitting outside of the gym and absorbing the sunshine before class and always just smiling away. Little did I know what all was happening in her life behind the many smiles and outgoing laughter that came from her each time I saw her. I believe we can all learn a lot from her and I feel blessed to have such a strong, yet sweet, person in my life. Thank you Laurence. Oh, and extra thanks for all the chocolates you always bring back from France for me!
Without further adieu, here's Laurence's story:

I have always been an exercise enthusiast. Any activity with fun and music attracts me. Music and group classes work for me because they are so motivating. Spin, zumba, bodyworks, step and yoga- you name it. I love to go for long walks with my friends and family when not working out.

Group classes also stimulate/trigger a competitive instinct inside of me. I feel the incredibly positive energy of the people around me. This energy is a "must" for me to stay "Happy go lucky".

What I love the most about boot camp is that each time I go I am part of a different group. I love meeting new people! We don't really speak about work so I go home more relaxed and I sleep better. I met my very good friend Jordan at step class and since, we have been partnering in a lot of group classes. She is now my workout buddy and I love it! We make plans every day and try to do as many classes as possible. Meeting Jordan and other super nice people at the gym is a major, major motivator for me to keep going.

As I said, I am a 'Happy go lucky" type of person. I have a very positive outlook on things, people and life in general. I consider myself to be well rounded. I am always down for a good laugh since it's not in my nature to take myself too seriously. Honestly, I don't think I am exceling in bootcamp. However, when I do bootcamp I feel stronger and I have more endurance for other classes. Burpees, Push-ups and Mountain Climbers are definitely not my favorite. I would rather do suicides (yep that tells you how much I don't love the other drills… ☺).

When I am in class or working out in the gym I find myself thinking about a lot. I end up thinking less at bedtime, which is a huge plus. Typically, working out puts me in a very happy, jovial mood. It energizes me; and I need all the energy I can get with my job because I have to wear so many different hats all day long. I am also able to maintain a decent weight (though it does fluctuate) by keeping my workout routine.

You really will see a change in your body and strength if you stick to a workout routine. I exercise an average of 5 days a week. I do about 3 classes weekly and on my days off (weekends) I typically do double classes (i.e. spin and power yoga or step and power yoga). I realize overdoing it is not good for me anymore. If I do not balance my workout activities, I find myself hurting, which down the road requires time off for recovery.

I have always had tons of energy. I have strong legs, maybe less strength in my arms. Power yoga and free weights have helped my arms to get stronger. I have to take time off frequently due to my work schedule or traveling/leisure schedule. I try to not take too much time off but sometimes it is inevitable. Getting older, I feel like I have to start all over again when I get back to the gym and often it takes me longer to get back in shape.

Life was healthy and balanced for the longest time. Then I was in a car accident in France with my dad while visiting back in March 2014. I feel like my health has gone downhill since then. My immune system has been down and I have been sick more than I ever have been this past year.

I have to watch what I eat to a certain extent. I cook everything I eat and try not to eat out too often. I treat myself on the weekends but during the week I watch my food and alcohol intake. I have to. I don't have one of those "great metabolisms." I love veggies and fruits. They are definitely part of my diet. I also make a lot of soups. My mom always made everything from scratch (she still does). My mom buys everything fresh from the markets. I try to live up to the same standard to a certain extent.

Recently, I was diagnosed with breast cancer. I went through double mastectomy surgery on Friday, August 28. I also had reconstruction breast surgery that day; at least the expanders', part one. I went in for another surgery in few months after. I was not afraid of what my appearance would be like. But I was concerned about the recovery time and possibly the lack of energy I might have after recovery. Not being able to be as active as I like to be and have been, and not being able to see the people I see on daily basis at the gym was most difficult for me. But now that I am back, I am so grateful to be *able to* invest in my health again.

I wouldn't be happy if I didn't fight for my health and my strength. If you want to make a positive change toward health and new friendships, go for it and don't give up. It may not be so great at first. You may think, "this is too hard" or that you look ridiculous. But you need to have perseverance. I am very tenacious by nature (the French and the Italian in me).

Exercising is so good for us and contributes to our wellbeing in general. Learn to really listen to how you feel. It is ok to push yourself and it is ok to give yourself some rest too. Some days are good some days are not so good. Learn to adapt your workout to who you are. If fitness is a part of your life, one light day or day off is not going to hurt you. You may just find that you love working out so much that you can't keep yourself away from it! You may, like me, find new friends and a reason to fight for life.

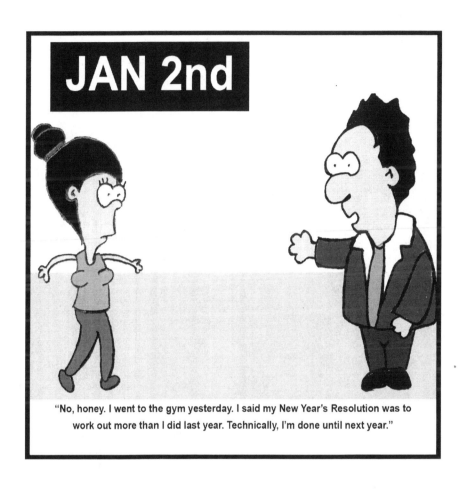

"No, honey. I went to the gym yesterday. I said my New Year's Resolution was to work out more than I did last year. Technically, I'm done until next year."

"The secret of change is to focus all of your energy, not on fighting the old, but on building the new."

- Socrates

SHAREEN

I'm happy to introduce my beautiful and sweet friend, Shareen. She's a 35 year-old, Bangladeshi-American woman with 2 children who also works as a software engineer. She loves to hike and is trying very hard to love running, too. She enjoys eating any food that is bad for her and she keeps a special place in her heart just for donuts. Shareen works hard in class but you can tell she works hard in everything that she does too. She once told me that she was going on a fast and I can't remember how long it was for but I want to say it was 6 weeks. I may be wrong about that but I know I'm right when I say she's extremely unique and definitely very disciplined in anything she decides to do. She also enjoys traveling when she gets the chance. I forgot to ask where her favorite place to travel to is but I'm going to guess anywhere outside of Arizona – especially during the scalding hot summer months (March – October). I'm very happy she shared her story and I know that she will strengthen many lives with it.
Without further adieu, here's Shareen's story:

I have never been a very athletic person. Growing up I never participated in any sports. Although I was not out of shape or overweight, I was not that physically strong either. I coasted through life until I hit my 30's and was faced with the biggest hurdle I have ever encountered. I found myself in a failing marriage with an almost two-year old. To top it off, I was 7 months pregnant. I was physically, mentally, and emotionally at the weakest I have ever been in.

At this place in my life, failure was not an option for me with two young children that depended on me for everything. So, I picked myself up and I rebuilt my life. I worked harder than I ever have at my job. I bought a new home for my little family. I found a job closer to home so I could better juggle a very demanding full-time career and still be there for my kids at every school event. And, I also joined a gym. I had not entered a gym in almost 5 years so it was incredibly intimidating at first. I did not know where to start, what exercises to do, or how to use the machines.

I started going to group fitness classes with two friends and that is how I discovered bootcamp. I found it was a great way to push myself physically, learn new exercises, and see some familiar faces. When I first started, I could barely make it through class. Slowly, as my endurance started to increase I found myself adding cardio exercises before the bootcamp classes. I started with 5 minutes on the elliptical machine, then 10 minutes, then running 2 miles before the class. I have since discovered a love for hiking and will find myself taking on 5-8 mile hikes on the weekends. I even take my children on smaller hikes with me on weekends when the weather is nice.

It has been 3 years now since I started the process of rebuilding my life and myself. Health and fitness has become an integral part of my life. At 35, I am physically stronger than I have ever been and I am not done. I live an incredibly full, hectic, and blessed life and I look to the gym as my "me" time. It is the one thing I do solely for myself. Working out and coming to the gym isn't about looking good or fitting into a smaller pair of jeans, it's about being the strongest I can be and continuing to grow stronger.

As a mom, I find it incredibly important to serve as a healthy role model to my children. I want to teach my children about the benefits of eating healthy food and living an active lifestyle. I do not want them to be motivated by vanity but by strength and resilience. Thank you, Robby, for being a part of that and for helping me grow.

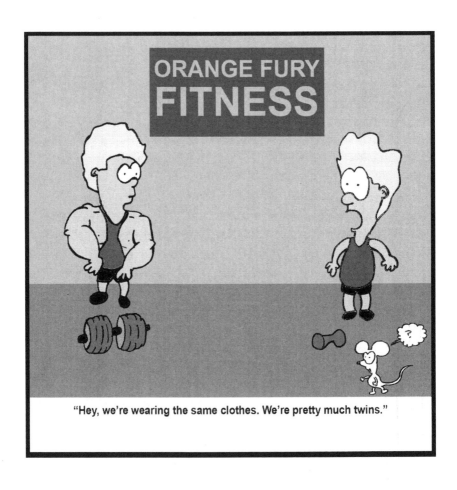

"A healthy outside starts from the inside."
- Robert Urich

ALLISON

Let me introduce you to my friend, Allison. She's a 37 year-old, teacher who's single with no kids. She lives in Mesa, Arizona. She is one of the stronger bootcampers in class, attending even though she recently broke her wrist. She forgets I can see everyone in the mirrors in class and I caught her doing one-armed knuckle burpees with the hand that was broken. Her favorite exercise in class is squat pulses and I'm willing to bet she's able to do more than a thousand in a row. She works out hard and sweats enough in class that she could end her training with another one of her passions...swimming. Allison shares some of my favorite foods. She loves Mexican food and her favorite cheat food is ice cream. One day, I'm going to challenge her to a burrito-eating contest where the loser has to pay for Cold Stone afterwards. She's tough but anyone who knows me knows that I already won. I'm always happy to see her at class as she brings great energy that makes me feel happy, as well as all those around her. Thank you for sharing your story!
Without further adieu, here's Allison's story:

For the last few years I have been really unhappy with my appearance. I had been working out on my own but was not seeing very many results. I was really frustrated with my lack of muscle tone and some specific body parts like my stomach and back. I wasn't completely out of shape. I felt like I was pretty strong actually, but did not have much muscle tone. I decided last year that the only way to change this was to do something about it.

So one year ago I really started working out hard. In the beginning, it was 1-2 times per week. I enjoyed taking BodyWorks (a total body weights class) and cycle as well as bootcamp. Now that I have gotten into bootcamp, I work out 2-5 times a week and don't feel good when I am unable to make it to class. It only took about a month for me to get hooked on exercise and want to make it a top priority.

I really enjoy the positive vibes and positive people in

Bootcamp. I feel that no matter what, I can always do whatever exercise is put in front of me. In the beginning, burpees, squat pulses and jump squats were too hard to complete but now I excel at them. Seeing this growth keeps me coming back. I also like the exercise variety every time I go. Everyone at bootcamp is at differing levels but both the instructor and participants always cheer you on, regardless of your level. Having friends to meet up with in class helps me stay more committed to myself and my fitness.

I have had 2 surgeries on my wrist and do not have full mobility. This makes some exercises more difficult, but my instructors give suggestions on other ways to try an exercise or a totally different exercise that works the same area. My wrists don't have to limit my workouts.

Now that working out in classes is a normal part of my life, I feel like I have a lot more energy at work and I can tell that I have more endurance in everything I do. Exercise has also made me open my eyes and really look at my diet: see how else I can help my body for the better. It also has helped me with relaxing after a stressful week or even day at work. None of these benefits are minor. Life is so much better when I make my own health a priority.

It's important to start somewhere when you want to see change in your life. Don't be intimidated by what bootcamp looks like from the outside, just try it! Try it for at least a month, and I can guarantee that if you push yourself, you will see results. You will always have people to cheer you on. If you believe, you can do anything!

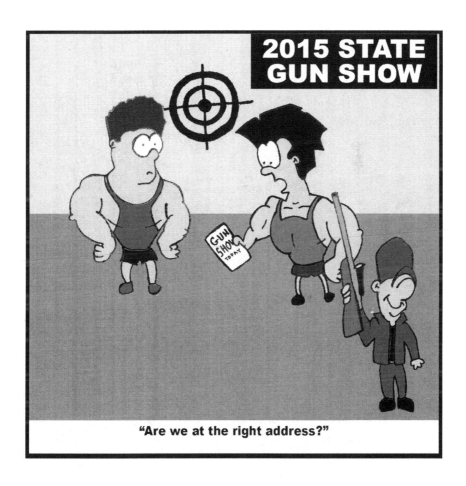

"You're in pretty good shape for the shape you are in."
- Dr. Seuss

PATRICIA

This next person I'm introducing to you makes me smile both inside and out just by her presence. She has a smile that lights up an entire building. Her name is Patricia and she is a 47 year-old, Hispanic female that works for the Phoenix Police Department. She is married with two sons, whom she preps healthy meals for every day. Patricia is also a certified Zumba instructor. Like I mentioned above, the one thing that stands out to me about her is her beautiful smile and her amazing energy. She claims to be 47 but you'd never guess it if you met her. She is always laughing and it's highly contagious to anyone around her. She does bootcamp, Zumba, and spends her time smiling and laughing. She has a wonderful sense of humor and she never fails to brighten my life and my mood. I'm blessed to have such an amazing person as a friend in my life. Thank you for sharing your story and for making this world a happier place.

Without further adieu, here's Patricia's story:

I've exercised consistently my entire life. There was a recent time that I was inconsistent working out due to illness (Thyroid Cancer and Hypercalcemia). I was diagnosed February 11, 2015. I lost a total of ten pounds and became weak. My symptoms included tingling, numbness, shortness of breath and dizziness. My doctors recommended that I take it easy for a while, which was hard for me. I was so anxious to pick up right where I left off.

On a good day, prior to getting sick, I would complete Bootcamp, along with a three hour Zumba session. Some days I would lift weights and then I would continue with cardio. I would go hike a mountain, then finish my day with a speed and agility class. Now, I focus on either cardio or weights or legs or Zumba. My husband and my older son are both fitness trainers and football kicking coaches. My son is also my very own personal trainer. He has taught me how to manage my form while lifting weights. I need the supervision, especially when it comes to a certain exercise that may strain my body. My twelve-year old son also knows the importance of exercise and he challenges me with treadmill and ab exercises.

I have attended Bootcamp classes at different gyms with trainers who solely belong to the gym and have no personal interest in watching their students succeed and learn and become stronger. This class is not like that. Approximately one year ago I walked into LA Fitness on Dobson and Warner and tried the Bootcamp class. The instructor was highly recommended from a friend of mine who had taken his taken his class before. After the one class, I was hooked. I loved the supervision that was given during the class, and I loved the way the stations were set up. I also loved all the positive energy that filled the class from the other students who were there. The music playlist was great.

Through my illness and after my treatment and receiving permission from my doctors to exercise again, I had one goal in mind: return to Bootcamp and my other exercise classes and get in the best shape of my life. I walked into Bootcamp with a smile on my face because I knew I was going to get a great workout.

I might be having a bad day, but after I finish my bootcamp class, everything seems so much better, and I feel stronger mentally and physically. Bootcamp helps me feel like myself again! My favorite exercise is (up/down) planks. My weakness has always been breathing through the exercise. This is something I really need to work on. I may not be the fastest or the strongest person in the room, but I'll be damned if I am not trying my hardest. For me, some days it's not about health or building muscle, it's just therapy. Bootcamp is not easy, but it's worth it!

My advice to others is: whatever you may be going through, please remember you are strong, you will get through it. If you can, get to Robby's Bootcamp class, I know you will leave class feeling GREAT!

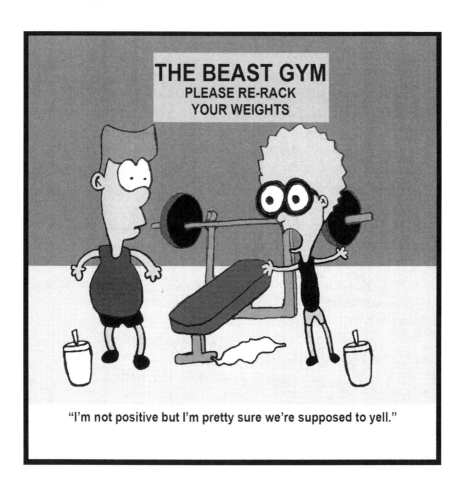

"It is health that is the real wealth and not pieces of gold and silver."

- Gandhi

MYCHAL

This next person I'd like to introduce is a true athlete and a good friend to many. His name is Mychal and he's 26-year old African-American who works as an International Product Specialist. Many things stand out about him both physically and characteristically. Physically, he's probably the fastest person in class and he jumps the highest. Anyone around him usually sees the bottom of his shoes whenever he jumps up. I once saw him jump so high that he decided to head-butt the basketball downwards through the hoop instead of just dunking it. Even though he's athletically talented, Mychal has compassion for just about everyone who's around him. It's one thing to be a nice person but it's a great thing to be genuinely caring for everyone. A fun fact about Mychal is his ability to eat a lot like I do. We went to Chipotle and he ordered quadruple meat on his burrito bowl because he was on a strict diet. Although some say I may have met my match, we shall see on the party pizza throw down between us the summer of 2016. Tickets go on sale soon!
Without further adieu, here's Mychal's story:

I started working out not very long ago...only when I started playing basketball in the second grade! Basketball is one of the great loves of my life so I have to keep in shape to perform on the court. Since I have been active all my life, my fitness level was pretty high before I started bootcamp classes. But my endurance was weak. I worked hard as a teen to get my speed and power, but knew I needed to up my stamina if I was going to be able to average the high level of points I wanted to at my games.

Before taking bootcamp I worked out 4 times a week at the gym. Back in May, a friend invited me to take a bootcamp class. I loved it. Now I work out 6 times a week and take bootcamp about 3 of the days. When I started, burpees were difficult, but thanks to my friend Angel pushing me, now I am great at them. I also have improved my jump in bootcamp. Most people around me get a few inches off the ground during jump squats. I get a few feet off the ground.

Exercising has had a substantial impact on my discipline, confidence and will power. Two years ago, I lost 40 pounds in 4 months. I have kept the weight off with exercise, both on the court and in the gym. I feel so much better about myself when I am fit, and bootcamp has helped me tone up and build more muscle. Other than the physical benefits of bootcamp, I enjoy the people the most! I have made close friends. The positive and energetic atmosphere is very captivating and inspiring. There are also great networking opportunities there.

Taking bootcamp has definitely impacted me mentally. I have gained a better sense of respect for myself, I wake up each day with more energy, and my nutrition has gotten much more appropriate. I was diagnosed with borderline diabetes when I was in 6th grade so what I eat matters. I am a meat lover though. I can grill a mean steak. Since starting bootcamp I have added veggies to my home cooked dinners. My more balanced diet has really increased my stamina, which has been proven a number of times on the basketball court.

I would encourage anyone to exercise, but especially to take bootcamps. Aside from the great people and amazing energy there, getting in the gym and working toward your goals will increase your discipline and will power. This benefits your work and personal life as well. Once you achieve your fitness goals, you quickly realize what you can accomplish outside of exercising, given you put in the same amount of work, time and dedication. I have big goals for my career and I "exercise" at work every day. Being fit and healthy, driven and disciplined only empowers me more. I live by Micheal Jordan's mantra: "I never feared or doubted my skills because I knew I put in the work."

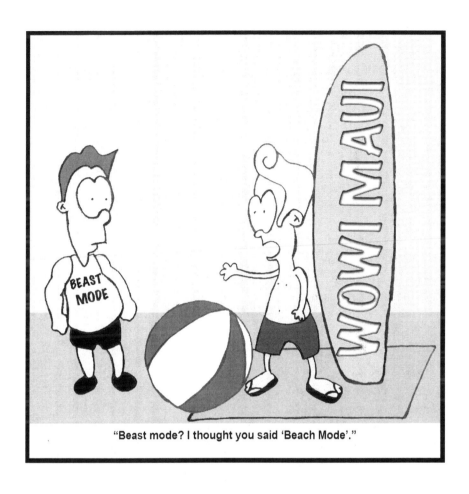

"Life is like a bicycle. To keep your balance, you must keep moving."

- Albert Einstein

BRITTNEY

I'm happy to introduce this next woman to everyone. Her name is Brittney and she is a 38-year old auditor from Mesa, Arizona. Although her favorite cheat food is pizza, Brittney has lost about 65 lbs in the last year. Many might be curious to what type of pizza she's been eating but I can tell you it's not the pizza, it's the other things she's been eating combined with how hard she's been pushing herself in her workouts. Brittney is inspiring more people than she knows just through her workouts in class, her amazing journey this past year, and by constantly spreading positive messages to others on her Facebook profile. I know her journey very well as weight loss has been a huge part of my own story. She's one to look up to when it comes to setting our minds to something, taking action, and never giving up and seeing it through. I'm very happy that she decided to be a part of this book and I'm very grateful that she is my friend.

Without further adieu, here's Brittney's story:

I feel like my fitness journey has been ongoing for my entire adult life. However, in the last year I got very serious about becoming a fit and healthy person. I realized that I had some very unhealthy habits and limiting beliefs about myself. I finally stopped feeding all the reasons I wasn't able to lose weight and be fit, all my limiting beliefs: "I've always been overweight," "I will have to buy all new clothes," "I have a thyroid problem," "It's not that bad," "I'm addicted to sugar," "I'm too old," etc. Finally, I just decided to go for it: just try and see what could happen. I thought, *if other people can do this, why not me?*

My goal was to lose 40 pounds. I decided I would eat clean and work out twice a day. No cheat days for me. I went cold turkey on sugar/sweets. I tracked my food and exercise in My Fitness Pal. I decided to really dedicate myself to the cause and just see what would happen....

Fitness classes at the gym were part of my daily routine. Being in a group setting really helped motivate me. Robby's

Bootcamp class on Wednesday was definitely a part of my weekly routine for the first 6-8 months. It was fun/challenging and over time I was able to see improvements. When I first started working out and coming to bootcamp, I felt like I was going to puke every time after doing suicides and burpees! I couldn't do more than 5 "real" pushups. Today, I can do suicides and burpees without feeling sick and actually enjoy them! And I can do lots of "real" pushups: it's awesome!

It wasn't long before the weight started coming off: I think within 6 weeks I had lost 20 pounds. This was motivation to keep going. When I hit my 40-pound weight loss around the holidays I got scared! I thought I was going to start gaining and doing the yo-yo thing I had always done. But I didn't want to; I decided to just keep going!!! I read that if you eat healthy and work out, your body will naturally settle at the weight it's supposed to be, so I decided to find out where that was. I have far surpassed any goals I set for myself. I'm in the best shape of my life and have done things physically I never thought I could do. I recently hiked 40 miles in 3 days in the Colorado Rockies! So grateful for my body being able to do this and carry me to such beautiful places!

I am especially grateful to the fitness instructors who show us how it's done. And who encourage us in classes, making fitness fun.

For me this was and still is much more than just a physical transformation. I believe that we are only truly healthy and whole when we work on ourselves from the inside out. I had to take a good hard look at what was driving my unhealthy lifestyle choices/patterns. I haven't got it all figured out yet, but I'm enjoying the journey and I know that the best is yet to come.

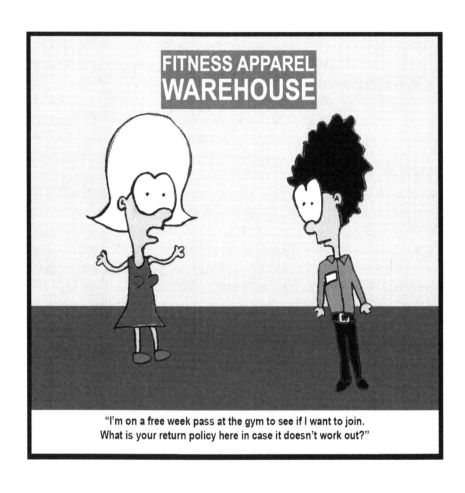

"The secret to getting ahead is getting started."
- Agathe Christie

AMBER

This next person I'm happy to introduce is Amber. She is a 32-year old stay-at-home mother from Phoenix, Arizona. She's loves to camp, eat chicken curry, and anything chocolate. Amber is small but has a huge personality and amazing sense of humor. Although, we don't talk as much in person as we do online, her posts on Facebook keep me laughing just about every day. Sometimes if I'm feeling a little down, I'll visit her page just to read what she's posted to lift my spirits back up. I believe she could have a great comedy career in blogging if she wanted to. I'm extremely happy that she attends my bootcamp class. I remember my first class that she took was one I held at the park, which is much more challenging and intense than my classroom format. She got through the class at the park and continued to come even after that. This says quite a bit about her commitment and priorities. Today, she's one to motivate others to come to class and I believe she'll be an inspiration to many all over the world. I'm very happy to have made a new friend and that she decided to be a part of this book.

Without further adieu, here's Amber's story:

Before I started working out, I spent almost two years pregnant and bedridden. I lost 20 pounds each pregnancy and I couldn't eat or drink anything without vomiting. I was weak, tired, and I had lost a lot of muscle.

I had always been active as a kid, teenager, and in my early 20's. But I got lazy and comfortable after I met my boyfriend (now husband). We started drinking a lot and didn't care about our health very much. After a couple of years, we were both 20 pounds heavier than when we first met. My husband had two health scares with alcoholic pancreatitis. I felt that I had to do something to motivate him to drink less and for both of us to start taking care of our bodies. The weight gain and health scares that I saw in others around me really motivated me to work out.

When I finally started taking bootcamp classes, I

thought the whole class was insane. I couldn't do any of it. I couldn't even make it through the warm up when I first started. When I finally did that, I found that I couldn't even do one girl push-up. Now, I can do about 40 of them. Even though it seemed impossible, I was hooked after the first class. I just couldn't believe how out-of-shape I had become so I bought a gym membership right away. Before bootcamp class, my workouts were jogging 3 nights per week and Total Gym (home workout machine) 4 nights per week. Now my workout consists of bootcamp 3-4 nights per week. If I miss class, I do similar workouts at home. I also try to walk or jog every day.

Exercise has changed my home life quite a bit. I have a lot more energy with my kids. My husband and I are closer now because I am much happier. We save a lot of money since we don't eat out nearly as much or buy alcohol. I am a much happier person now that exercise has become such a big part of my life.

What I love most about bootcamp class is that energy and motivation that everyone gives each other. Everyone is friendly, the class is fun, the music is great, and it's, overall, just very motivating. I think we wouldn't have a class like this without such an awesome, funny, and caring fitness instructor.

From my experience, in order to continue and succeed in weight loss and fitness, you have to find a workout that you enjoy doing. You also have to have motivation and want to do it. I've been doing bootcamp since May 25th this year and so far I've lost 20 lbs. And the best thing: I find that I can force myself to show up to bootcamp completely tired and leave class happy, feeling great, and full of energy. I love it.

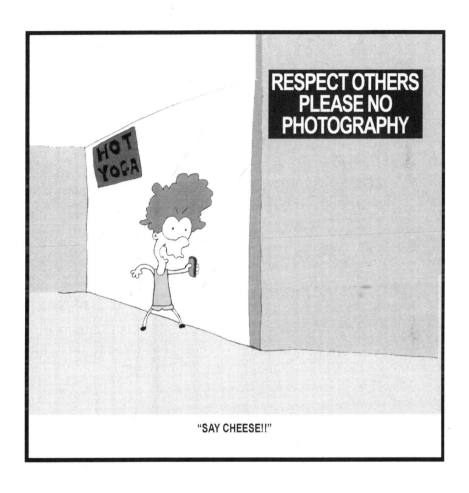

"No matter how much it gets abused, the body can restore balance. The first rule is to stop interfering with nature."
 - Deepak Chopra

C.D.

This next person I'm introducing is a superstar of a person. Not just in her workouts but in real life. She has more friends than I see people have. The reason for it is because of the type of friend she is. It's not just her sweet personality. She is a down-to-earth real person who isn't afraid to share her own thoughts and opinions with her friends. People are very drawn to her and whenever you talk to her, you feel like you're talking to your best friend. I'm happy she shared her story for this book and I'm extremely grateful for her kindness and compassion in our friendship.
Without further adieu, here's her story:

Growing up with my bipolar, manic-depressive mother, there was no emphasis on anything besides the religion she poured herself into. No school and no physical activity. The few times I did go to school I loved P.E. It was the only thing I really loved.

The things I experienced in those formative years with my abusive mother have always stayed with me. By age 13 I was a total wreck and knew if I didn't leave I would eventually end my life. I had watched my mother attempt suicide several times and it seemed the most likely direction I was headed. I contacted my older sister and begged for help. My father called a week later and spoke to my mother. A month later I was on a plane to go live with him. That month of waiting was one of the worst months of my life but, obviously, I survived it.

The weekend I went to live with my dad, step-mom and sister was the Honolulu Marathon. My father was stationed in Hawaii and had always been a very active person. I dare say that watching my dad and step-mom complete the marathon gave me the most incredibly happy chills and changed my life.

I wanted to run a marathon. I wanted to run, period. Living in Hawaii was the perfect place to start and my dad was all for it. I started running with him pretty regularly and by the time I got to high school I joined cross country and track. My world had changed. I still carried all the pain from my past, but when I was running and around my teammates I was completely happy. I started to do road races, actually including some cycling events. All aspects of my life improved. Sadly, I began experiencing severe pain in my feet and knees and had to quit running my senior year.

Many years later, as a new wife and mother, the pain returned. My baby was only 4 months old and I was not even running. Two long years passed before I was diagnosed with severe, progressive Rheumatoid Arthritis. It was so severe, it destroyed the bones in my hands in less than 5 years. By age 26 my rheumatologist did a bone scan, revealing that my bones had deteriorated to the point of osteopenia. He had never seen anyone my age that bad. This was when I realized I needed to get back to exercising.

Enter again running. I had to try to "fix" myself so I started power walking and jogging. I found that more often than not, the days I ran I became more comfortable. I was still suffering from RA but my exercise world opened back up. My bones slowly but surely improved as well. From ages 30-40 I ran; completing 5 full marathons, 10 half marathons, countless smaller races and, well, a divorce.

Today, like everyone, I have my personal struggles with life and relationships. The one and only constant (other than RA) is my commitment to myself. I don't run anymore due to heel spurs but I work out almost daily. My body needs to move.

I have had active RA for 26 years now. I fully believe that I would be in far worse physical condition if I didn't have my love affair with exercise. More importantly though, is the healing mentally I have experienced. I can't express how much it keeps me on track emotionally. I honestly feel exercise and the community it brings saved my life.

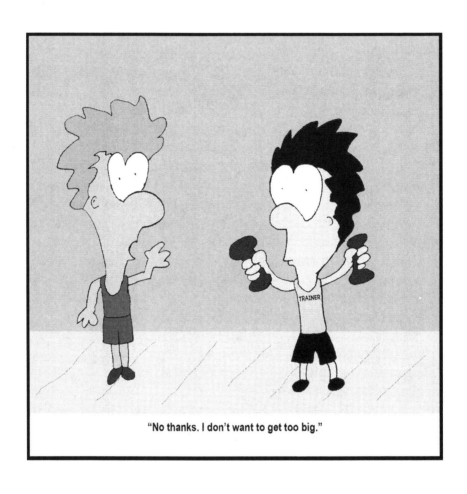

"I always wanted to be in the health and wellness business. I try to encourage people to live a healthy lifestyle."
                                                    - Mark Wahlberg

ANTHONY

This next person I'd like to introduce you to is Anthony. He's a 28-year old Asian who works as a web developer. His favorite food is sushi and his cheat food of choice is anything with carbs since he's been strict on his carb intake. Anthony enjoys playing basketball and watch movies in his free time. One thing that stands out about Anthony is the fact that he looks like a movie star. If you put him in a suit and a pair of sunglasses on him, people might line up to get autographs. The question is: would he sign them or not? I guess that all depends on how many carbs he's allowed himself to have that day. Actually, he's one of the nicest people you'd ever meet and I'm sure he'd sign an autograph for you...even if you didn't ask politely. I'm happy to be his friend and I look forward to seeing him in a movie I may or may not write very soon.

Without further adieu, here's Anthony's story:

When I was around 18 years old I was a really skinny 130 pounds, standing 5'11." I was pretty stressed out in life. I started lifting weights and playing basketball and realized they were a great outlet. I started seeing positive change, mentally and physically. I never watched what I ate and by the time I was 23 I started getting a chubby tire around my waist. That prompted a change toward healthier eating.

Now I am 28 and currently work at home. Being sedentary drives me insane sometimes since I like to move a lot. I've always been an on-again off-again exercise person, but currently I am in my longest active stretch: over 2 years! I usually work out 3-6 days a week, so when a friend introduced me to bootcamp about a year ago, I thought, why not try something new at the gym. He seemed to really love the class. Bootcamp really helps me release pent up energy from having to sit in my office for so many hours.

The hardest challenge to working out is consistency and discipline. The leg exercises in bootcamp were the toughest part for me in the beginning – my legs were skinny and weak. But the community of class, the energy I take from it, the confidence and stress relief I feel have made the challenge worth it. I have seen a huge gain in my endurance since taking bootcamp. My legs are also much stronger now. I have a strong determination to push past my limits. This comes alive both in class, the gym floor and on the basketball court.

The community I am a part of is a great part of bootcamp. We get together to eat after class sometimes, we hang out after class sometimes and laugh about the stations that were hard for us that night. The people that go to class understand my love of being active and the high that I get from feeling healthy and strong. I am now 35lbs heavier than my once 18-year old skinny self, and that's without wearing a tire around my waist!

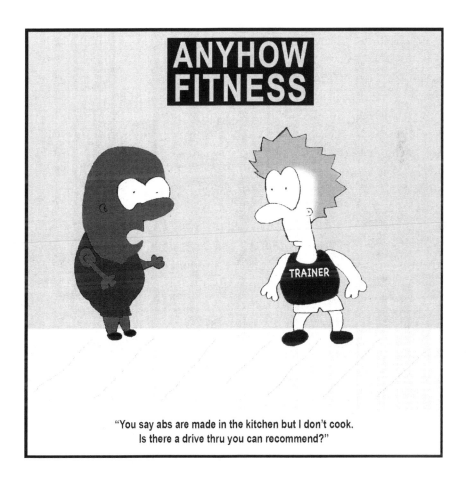

"I think that age as a number is not nearly as important as health. You can be in poor health and be pretty miserable at 40 or 50. If you're in good health, you can enjoy things into your 80s."

- Bob Barker

MELISSA

I'd like to introduce Melissa. She is one of the happiest people I know and always has a smile on her face – probably because some of her favorite things to do are going to the beach, spending happy hour with her husband and, of course, exercising. She's 49 years old with 5 kids and works as an executive assistant but you'd swear she was 20 with no kids just by her looks and how much energy she has in class. She shares some of my favorite foods (and cheat foods), which are Mexican food, pizza and pizzookies from Oreganos. But, she tries to keep it under control by eating spinach salad just about every day. I'm always happy to see Melissa when she comes to class as she brings such good, positive energy with her that makes not just myself but for everyone around her feel happy. I'm so happy she shared her story and that she is someone I can call my friend.

Without further adieu, here's Melissa's story:

My journey in exercise started when I was young, as a teenager. However, even though I love running, I just ran my first full marathon only a couple of years ago. I loved the feeling of completing such a significant goal. My motivation comes from seeing the level of commitment my husband gives to fitness. I also want to set a good example for my kids.

I've always tried to workout 5 days per week. Since taking Robby's bootcamp and cycle classes, my level of fitness has really increased. However, it wasn't always easy. When I first started bootcamp, burpees seemed impossible to me. Now, they're pretty easy and I'm also much better at jump roping now. I love the positive effects that exercise has on me. I have the feeling of doing something good for myself and it keeps me feeling young.

My favorite part about bootcamp is that I really enjoy the camaraderie, meeting awesome people, and challenging myself physically. I also love the feeling of motivation that exudes throughout the room. It's a big stress reliever for me and I find that I'm generally just a better person when I exercise.

If I could offer any advice to someone it would be that it's never too late to start exercising and don't be afraid to go outside of the box. I can remember when I couldn't jog around the block but with discipline and training I ran my first marathon at the age of 48. I would encourage others to mix up their exercise routine and try new challenging exercises. Pinterest is a great source for me when I look for new exercises to try. I believe it doesn't matter what age or level of fitness you are at, there are always challenging exercises out there.

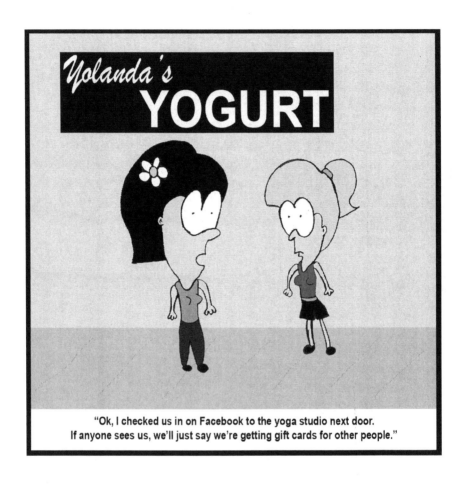

"To keep the body in good health is a duty, otherwise we shall not be able to keep our mind strong and clear."
                                                    - Buddha

Fang Ye

This next person I'm introducing happens to be a really close friend. I've known her since I taught my first class. Her name is Fannie (English version) and she is from Southeast China. Whether or not she knows this, I've seen her motivate hundreds of people just by her playful pushiness, sweet personality, and endless energy. Sometimes I would teach 12 or 14 classes in a week and Fannie would be at every single one of them, ready to go. She would also meet me every morning before class and run bleachers with me, often times showing up 30 minutes early just to get a head start. She has 2 boys and I believe one of her favorite things in life, besides exercising, is eating. I remember the first time we hung out and got dinner, she ordered about 12 different entrees and we shared them all. I've never been so full in my life and I had left overs for days. There are many positive things I can say about her but too much for an introduction. I do know that friends like her are one-of-a-kind and even though I'm her instructor, she equally has motivated me and makes me a better person. I'm more than blessed to have her in my life.

Without further adieu, here's Fannie's story:

Hello, my name is Fang Ye and I am from Southeast China. I have been in the U.S. for about 20 years and I have two lovely boys. They are my pride because they are much more intelligent than I am. I think I'm old enough to be your big sister.

I love reading because I believe reading enriches and fulfills my life. If I really have to pick one cheat food I would like to say pita chips; they are so tasty and crunchy. I am addicted to food. Eating is the joy of my life. For a while, I felt I lacked energy and for some reason I was always getting sick so I thought maybe working out would help me feel better about myself. Since 2007, I have been taking cycle, yoga, bodyworks, and bootcamp classes at the gym every morning after I drop off my boys at school.

Robby Wagner's bootcamp saved me from a crazy trip at the Grand Canyon in May of this year. I started taking his bootcamp class from the first day he began teaching at Dobson and Warner club, two years ago. I still clearly remember his first class. There were only 6 people in the class, but he was fine with it. Robby meticulously set up six stations. Before the class began, Robby patiently explained every exercise we were going to do. Throughout the whole class, he focused on encouraging every one of us, motivating us, and making sure we were using the correct form. We were so impressed by his passion, and the class was intense and fun. From then on, I have been taking his bootcamp classes as much as I can.

Robby's bootcamp class has grown much bigger and become more and more popular. Now we have 30 to 60 people in each class and 8 stations instead of 6. After taking Robby's bootcamp for over two years, I feel much more energized and strong. On May 30th of this year, I went hiking with my friends at the Grand Canyon. I feel strong and confident. I went ahead of my friends and I missed the trail that was supposed to take me back up. I ended up continuously hiking from 9:30am to almost 11:00pm. After the trip was over, I lost five toenails. When asked how I made it, my answer was "bootcamp saved me". The training from his class built my body, spirit, and willpower to keep going.

Besides physical benefits from going to the bootcamp classes I started to think more positively and make great friends with same interests. We motivate and encourage each other while exercising. I have also made great progress in terms of strength, like going from not being to do a single pushup to knocking out 25 pushups in just a minute. But most importantly, now I can eat whatever I want and whenever I want without feeling guilty because I know I'm going to work it off during classes.

If I can offer advice to anyone that's reading this: do not give up, keep going no matter what; you will see the difference.

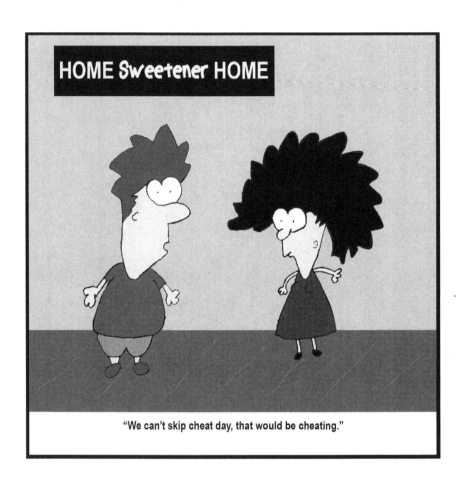

"Our bodies are our gardens - our wills are our gardeners."
- Shakespeare

BRE

I'm pleased to introduce my next friend, her name is Breanne but we call her Bre. She's a beautiful, single 31-year old Health Coach from Pinetop, Arizona and one of the sweetest and caring people you may ever meet. She currently has over 700 pairs of yoga pants (all different colors), which equates to about one pair for each workout she does in a year. You'd never guess by her fancy nails that she could do so many non-assisted pull-ups and make it look easy. I once saw her do 50 pull-ups in a row but I wasn't counting. Even though her profession is to help company staff in the corporate setting with their wellness, Bre helps many people in class or out on the floor with exercises and nutrition tips just out of the passion and kindness she has for helping others in their journey. I know it may come to a surprise to many but she occasionally treats herself to chips and salsa or cake as a cheat meal. Her favorite food is Chipotle. Oh wait, that's someone else. Her favorite food is sushi. I'm blessed to have such a beautiful person inside and out in my life that I can call my friend. She is one that many look up to or reach out to and she never lets them down. She changes the world every day and I'm very happy she's part of this book.

Without further adieu, here's Bre's story:

Exercise has always been a huge part of my life. Ever since I can remember it has ALWAYS been a part of me. I started out loving to run as a kid. I was a fast runner and all the boys would want to race me. I thought it was so fun to beat them. That turned into me being really fast and quick in soccer, which lead to track.

One of our classes in high school was weight lifting. It taught us the different muscles and the importance of lifting weights to be stronger. The process of getting stronger and what that in turn did for my self-esteem fascinated me.

When I first went to college I was terrified to gain the "freshman 15." I started working out and running even more to avoid gaining weight. It took me many years to realize that I was working out for completely the wrong reasons. Now I work out to feel better. My goal when I work out is to be the best me for that workout. I feel that if you put those negative demands on yourself (fear of weight gain) it is much harder to love what you are doing. In this scenario, you are working out of fear instead of to better yourself. There are so many positive qualities I have taken away from sports, running and working out. I loved how sports shaped me as a person. It taught me self-discipline and a hard work ethic. It taught me how to be part of a team and to have others' interest in mind at all times. That same mentality I have taken into my adult life.

Playing sports and being physically active has always been my constant. I have always relied on being physically active to be my therapy in a sense. When I am sad, depressed, stressed etc, I work out harder. It truly has gotten me through some of my hardest times in life. What I know for sure is this: I feel the absolute prettiest and most confident after I finish a hard workout. I feel as if I can conquer the world and that right there is priceless.

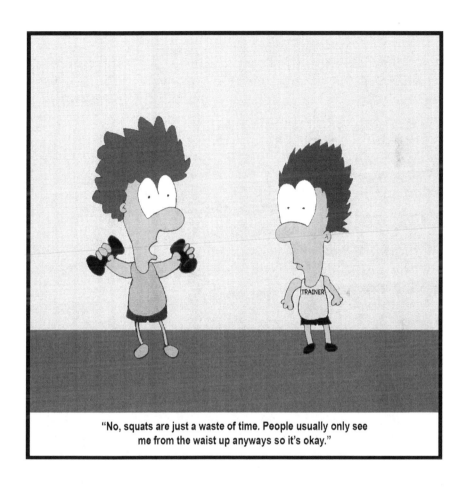

"I feel pretty good. My body actually looks like an old banana, but it's fine."

- Mike Piazza

LOUIS

I'm happy to introduce this next guy to you. His name is Louis and he's a 46-year old, African-American from Iowa that works in U.S. Customs. He's married with 2 kids and his favorite cheat food is warm Dutch apple pie with ice cream. Louis is in tremendous shape and is actually one of the most physically fit people I know. I also know that he runs marathons so it shocks me to see how fast he sprints, as well. Usually, I see one or the other but he's exceptional at both. I think if marathons had a track where people could go bet on runners, I would, without a doubt, put my money on him. It's really an honor that he takes my classes and expresses the benefits he gets from them considering the shape he's in. I'm very happy that we became friends and maybe one day we'll set up a race against each other and sell tickets to it. We'll take the ticket sales and go buy the biggest Dutch apple pie with ice cream that money can buy!
Without further adieu, here's Louis's story:

Some people might look at my fitness level and be intimidated. After all, I run marathons and often do "two-a-days," that is, running in the morning and hitting the gym for bootcamp at night. So here's the wild little secret: I didn't really start exercising until age 42. I was tired of how my clothes fit and wanted to get healthy. Occasionally I would go to the gym, but I had high cholesterol and certainly wasn't fit. Mentally I felt really out of shape, and getting out of that mindset would be my biggest challenge. All exercises can at times seem impossible, even now that I have been working out for three years. But the progress is undeniable, so I keep investing in my health.

My wife inspired me to start running after she ran her first half marathon four years ago. I started running short races and soon wanted to train for longer ones. I worked up to marathons and have now participated in several races, including the PF Chang Phoenix and Las Vegas Half marathon, the Phoenix half marathon, and the Pat Tillman marathon. In

2014 I had worked myself to such a level that I was able to run the NYC Marathon.

In the beginning, I started exercising 2-3 days a week. Within six months I was a junkie. Now I run 4-5 times a week in the mornings and add bootcamp in a few nights a week. Taking class has made me stronger. I see improvements in my running endurance and my attitude toward fitness stays positive because of class. I really like the community of bootcamp. I get motivation in my groups as we work through the stations together and I also encourage other people to exercise and run. I have made friends through class, unique friendships that are built on the common goal of wanting to push ourselves to be better.

I am happier now that I am in excellent shape and have made fitness such a big part of my life. Who could have imagined that I would *start* running marathons in my late 30s? You never know what you are capable of doing until you try! Not only do I look better in my clothes, but I feel more confident and have taken control of my health. No plans to retire from the fitness life any time soon.

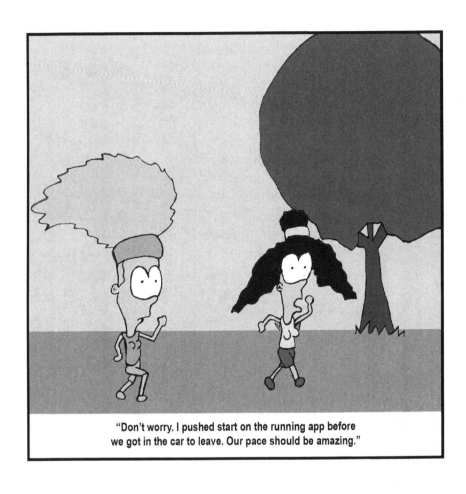

"The part can never be well unless the whole is well."
- Plato

ANGEL

This next person is someone I consider a dear, close friend of mine. Her name is Angel and she is one most of the time. Although she looks about 17, she's a 39 year-old single Mexican female whose favorite food is spaghetti. Her favorite exercises are burpees, running, and more burpees. She enjoys scrapbooking to relax from the 100+ miles she runs each month and reading to balance out the 10+ visits to the gym to lift weights each day. When she's not at the gym, running up a mountain, or training for a marathon, she can be found either trying on pink workout gear or eating ice cream while balling up her fists while yelling, "more burpees, more burpees, more burpees!" Don't be fooled by this small girl, her nickname is Princess Beast Mode for a reason.
Without further adieu, here's Angel's story:

I started exercising because at age 32 I had a difficult time running a simple 2 miles. I thought to myself, *at 32, this should not be this hard.* It was that day I decided to train and run a half marathon. I did not have any previous physical or medical conditions.

Once I started running and training for my first half marathon, which turned into training for a full marathon, I fell in love with exercising. The adrenaline rush from crossing the finish line of a marathon is like none other. I ran my first marathon in January 2011 and then went on to run four more that year. I could not get enough of that rush. Since then I have run a total of nine marathons.

Before I started Bootcamp I was in good shape. My number one strength was cardio because I am a marathon runner. My weakness was lack of strength. I could run forever but when it came to lifting weights, I definitely needed some muscle. I still work out 6-7 days a week but before starting bootcamp I only ran those days. Aside from bootcamp, I run and lift weights. I also do one workout in the morning and one at night. Adding weight lifting to my workouts has helped my running tremendously.

There wasn't an exercise in Bootcamp I felt was impossible. Burpees and push-ups seemed hard but not impossible. Now they are my two favorite stations in class. I love to challenge myself by doing different variations of each that make them harder.

My favorite things about Bootcamp are the different ways each exercise can be modified for each person. Each person can work at whatever fitness level she/he is comfortable. There is no trying to compete or keep up with other people in the class. You can challenge yourself as an individual; trying to do more of one exercise in the second round than you did in the first. No one has to know but you.

I also like to cycle for those very reasons too. No one knows what you are doing on the bike but you. You can ride at your own pace. Make the workout your own. In the end, that is what exercise is all about. It should be what you like, enjoy, and is best for your body.

After starting Robby's class, I've made some new friends that share my love of fitness. We get together outside of class too. We share our lives with each other. They motivate me to keep exercising. They have become people I lean on when times get hard and they have become people I want to share my happy times with first. I also schedule my day around my workouts/runs. My friends outside of my fitness family do not understand this. I often hear, "You can skip just one workout." At the fitness level I am at now, no I cannot. Exercise has become my number one priority. Without it, I find it hard function during the day. It has become something I need and crave for my overall wellness. In that respect, I do not see many of friends outside of my fitness family. I am perfectly fine with that. My fitness family surrounds me with positivity and motivation for more than just my workouts/runs.

The positive effects of exercise have been my ability to handle stress and keep me in a better mood throughout the day. I know that if I am having a bad day, I can count on my workout/run to make me feel better. On the opposite side, a good day leads to a great workout/run.

My energy level has also been heightened. I do not feel as tired and worn down by mid-afternoon anymore like I did before I started exercising. When I am tired, my workout/run re-energizes me as well. It is hard to explain the power that exercise has on your mind and body but once you feel it, there is nothing else like it. You want to keep that feeling as long as you can. You will do just about anything to make it keep coming back.

The advice I would give other people when trying to find a passion in exercise and fitness is this: make it your own. Find something you like to do. Running, hiking, swimming, weight lifting, Zumba, whatever that is – do it! Ignore all of the trendy things other people are doing. Find what works for your body, not what everyone else is doing. Second, learn to like the word diet. Diet is not a bad taboo word. It simply means, what you eat every day. If you like what you eat every day, great. As long as what you are eating is good for your body and mind. There is no shame in eating a cheeseburger and fries once in a while. Enjoy a scoop of ice cream with hot fudge, just not every day. Once you find a diet that works for you, it will become your lifestyle. That is the goal, to make diet and exercise part of your lifestyle. Last, I would tell people to not be so hard on themselves. So you had two cheat days instead of one. So you missed one workout. That really is ok, just make sure to get back on that horse. Remember, you are trying to make this part of your lifestyle. Doing that is not easy. It will not happen overnight or in a month or two. Keep at it, it will happen.

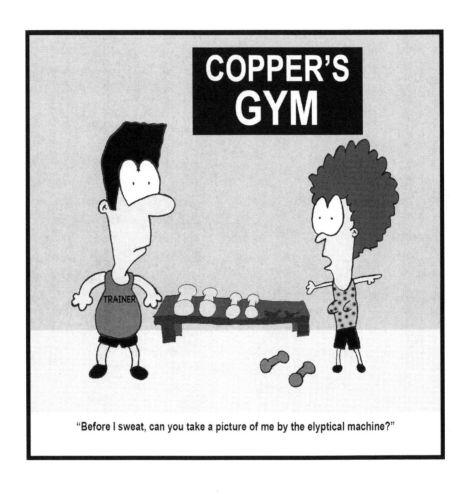

"There is no easy way out. Believe me, if there were, I would have bought it. And it would be one of my favorite things."
                                                        - Oprah Winfrey

JANE

It's my pleasure to introduce my good friend and someone I care for very much, Jane. If you saw her, you'd never guess she is 51 and single with 3 grown children. She's an elementary school teacher, which fits her well with her sweet personality. She is also one of the strongest people who take my class. One thing that really stands out in class is her ability to do military style push-ups and make them look so easy. Even though she's pretty small in size, she's stronger than most of the men in that area and it's an awesome thing to see in person. I first found out that we both share a lot of similar tastes for food when we ran into each other at Costco loading up on my favorite organic vegan protein. She must've had a hundred tubs loaded into her cart before they tried to make her put some back to share with other shoppers. Luckily, I just did triceps that day and I flex intimidated them to go bother other shoppers. I'm very happy that I can call Jane my friend. Anyone that knows her will tell you the same. She's as strong and dedicated to fitness as she is sweet and beautiful. Thank you for being my friend!

Without further adieu, here's Jane's story:

I have to begin by saying I don't have a story about *starting* an exercise program as I have been pretty active my whole life. I grew up on a farm and was outside working since I can remember. I still feel a sense of satisfaction and happiness when I do hours of yard work on the weekend. As far as exercising goes, I've gone through several phases throughout my life. I went to a small school in rural Iowa and was able to participate in several sports every year in school. When I was in college, it was about losing weight. I worked out to aerobic exercise videos in my apartment as joining a gym was not in my budget. Then I met a guy that got me into running. I became addicted and couldn't stand going a day without it. I quickly lost the 'freshman 15' pounds I had gained.

As life went on, I had 'distractions' that took me away from running, like moving, getting married, having children, working, etc. I finally decided I wanted to run a marathon to get me running consistently again. I hadn't run a race outside of high school track, but I decided to go for it. My strength has always been dedication and endurance. I checked out a book from the library and planned out my training schedule. I stuck to it and did every bit of training by myself. I did short runs during the week after work and long runs on the weekend. The running not only helped my physically, but mentally as well. My marriage wasn't working and the training was very therapeutic. Finishing the 26.2 miles at age 41 was a highlight in my life.

After the marathon, I kept running, but I wanted to mix it up a bit as my knees were feeling the wear and tear. I took a yoga class and loved how it made me feel. I loved it so much more than I thought I would. I read many books and I actually took courses and became certified to teach children's yoga. Next, I started going to the gym to lift weights. I just couldn't stick to it. It was boring to me. Then I took my first cycle class and loved it. It was such a great cardio workout and it was low impact so didn't affect my knees. I started going 3 times a week or more on top of yoga and running. I was addicted. I even got my own spin bike to use at home. I also bought a mountain bike and did that as well as swimming. I did all of that for several years.

Then my husband of 23 years and I divorced and I decided to start taking different classes at the gym to mix things up. I heard about Robby's bootcamp from a friend. I went one time and was addicted. I loved the intensity of the cardio, the music, meeting new people, but more than that, I loved the strength exercises. Finally, I had found a way I could use weights (and my body weight) for upper body strength and stick to it because it was fun! The thing that was the most difficult for me in the beginning were the pushups. I couldn't do more than a few without dropping to my knees. I knew that my upper body was my weakness, so I always put the most into that type of station/challenge. Now I can do 30+ regular/military pushups without stopping. I can see a difference in my arms that I've never seen before.

If I could inspire anyone to achieve better health/fitness, my advice would be to try different things until you find something you enjoy. Start by doing what you can. Try to put more into your areas of weakness instead of avoiding those areas, and keep going!

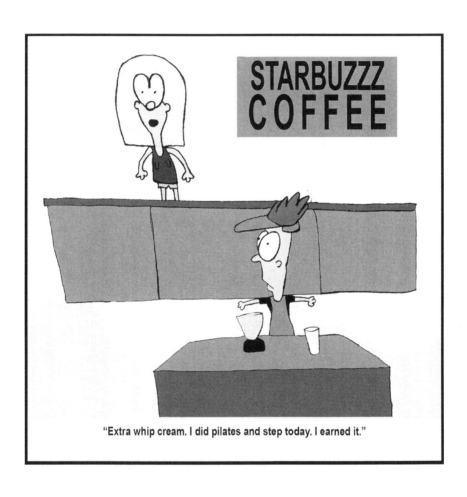

"A good laugh and a long sleep are the best cures in the doctor's book."

- Irish Proverb

JAMIE

Let me introduce you to Jamie. She is a 34-year old female from Las Vegas, Nevada who may or may not gamble and works as an administrative assistant for a homebuilding construction company. She has 1/64 Choctaw blood in her and 63/64 pale, white blood to the fullest. She married her high school sweetheart and he married her back. So, both officially married their high school sweethearts, at the same time and on the same day, in front of the same audience and with the same hecklers. They have a 15-year old son together and she's also a stepmom of an 11-year old daughter. When I pulled out the calculator, she said that's a story for another time and we shared a nice snorting laugh. Jamie enjoys going to rock concerts but not so much operas or piano recitals. Her favorite foods are burritos and pizza. I suggested she try pizzarritos and she asked where they have them but I didn't know...but I lied anyways and said Chipotle has them. I asked what her favorite exercise was and she said group fitness classes, in which she proceeded to pantomime them as I guessed. They were, in no particular order except for how I decided to write this out: bootcamp, kickboxing, yoga and Zumba. I'm excited for you to read her story and I'm thankful that we've become friends!

Without further adieu, here's Jamie's story:

Fitness was never a word used when I was growing up. Exercise? Yeah, right! Diet? ... Ummm, no. It wasn't until after I had my son that I began to worry about my weight and health. I was 20 years old and had gained 75 pounds during pregnancy. That was 15 years ago, and honestly, I'm only a few pounds short of where I was then, but the amazing energy and happiness I have now are a direct result of never giving up.

These days I don't worry about my weight and health. Worrying is stressful and stress does bad things to your body and mind. I'm not saying I don't care. Of course, I am mindful of my weight and have goals to continue to get that number on the scale down, but I have the peace of mind knowing that I am finally on the right track.

Over the last five years, my weight has dramatically fluctuated within a range of 100 pounds. How is that even possible? It's unbelievable even to me. So, this is how it happened:

In 2010, after working out and trying to eat healthy the whole year before - and having limited success, I heard about HCG. I was desperate to try something different and thought I needed quick results or I was going to give up. So, I did tons of research and ended up ordering from an online pharmacy and mixing this stuff myself. I injected myself with this hormone every day. I know-crazy, right?!

I followed the protocol strictly for the first 40 days and had great results, if you only consider the number on the scale. I did another round and ended up 55 pounds lighter than my initial weigh-in. Now, that sounds awesome, but what you don't know is how I felt while restricting myself to a mere 500 calories a day-everyday. During this process, I hadn't learned anything about proper nutrition. I certainly didn't create a healthy relationship with food. Needless to say, these results weren't sustainable. And this is where the 100 pounds comes in. I eventually gained back all of the weight I lost, plus an additional 45 pounds, ending up at a number that scared me so badly, it would change the course of my wellness journey.

I knew I had to get back to the basics. So, at the beginning of 2014, I limited my calorie intake and got myself back into the gym. Within a couple months, I began to feel better. I hadn't realized how much I was missing in my life. I had been on auto-pilot for years but didn't notice until I started to come out of the fog.

I found a solution to help me create the healthy relationship with food that had been lacking in my previous attempts. I now feel energy, balance, happiness, and confidence that everyone should experience in life.

After the HCG disaster, I found a bootcamp class that met up in a park. That really built up my belief in myself and my capabilities. It also made me understand that people will not judge me, but rather cheer me on as I try to get fit. From there, I began going to LA Fitness and found Yoga. This was a new experience to me because up until then, I thought working out had to be fast-paced and hectic in order to work. Yoga slows it down while still challenging me.

I took my first bootcamp class with Robby in May 2015. Getting back into group fitness helped me remember how much fun exercising can be. Working my butt off in a room full of people doing the same workout is a tremendous motivation to me. There are people of different ages and fitness levels and working hard with them, I feel like I am accomplishing something worthwhile.

My healthier relationship with food has everything to do with finding Isagenix. With their products, I have found help in meal planning (which I am horrible at) because the nutrition shake is equivalent to 3 plated, organic meals. I wouldn't even know where to begin if I wanted to buy, prepare, cook, and eat that much food and keep it up for very long. The energy and sense of well-being I feel when I am eating more balanced and healthy is priceless. Isagenix was for me personally, the catalyst that brought me out of my funk. The positive change in my diet partnered with exercise has awakened my dreams.

I have come to understand that I am directly responsible for my outcome. No one is going to exercise or eat for me. It's up to me. It always has been. Doing the work it takes to release this much weight is a little easier when surrounded by a group of people who are doing the work with you. I don't just go to a class at a gym when I'm in one of Robby's classes, I become part of a community of people that come together to work, motivate and inspire one another.

I can do this and so can you! Wherever you are in your journey, always remember to strive for progress over perfection. You may not know everything about everything, but getting out there and doing the work consistently will get you there. Strive on!

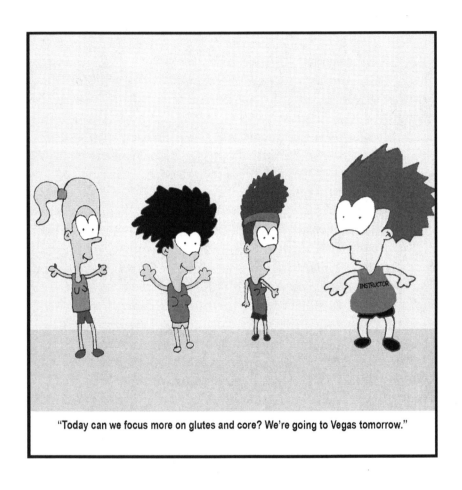

"Today can we focus more on glutes and core? We're going to Vegas tomorrow."

"Every accomplishment begins with the decision to try."
- Gail Devers

JEFF

This next friend I'm introducing has a true love for running and all things fitness related. His name is Jeff and he's a 68-year old Polish Catholic man from Brooklyn, New York. He's full of humor and his favorite Polish joke is that he's a Polish Physician/Anesthesiologist, which he tells patients right before they go into surgery. Jeff is one of those people who are just full of life all the time. He enjoys hiking, kayaking, playing the trumpet, big band music concerts, fountain pens, cars, and painting. For exercise, he loves running, hiking, cycling, bootcamp and boxing. One thing that stands out to me about Jeff is that he loves anything that allows him to jump. He enjoys jumping high and he enjoys jumping far, just like a frog. He also enjoys his runs, which he pretty much does daily. It's not rare that he comes to class after an 8-10 mile run to finish off his training for the day. Jeff has one son, one nephew, and one BMW – all of which he loves very much. With all of his training, I asked what his one and only favorite cheat food was and he told me pizza, chocolate, ice cream, and cookies. These may not be everyone's cheat food of choice but it certainly are mine most of the time. I appreciate Jeff's friendship very much and I know that his energy and commitment is contagious to all those around him.

Without further adieu, here's Jeff's story:

My motivation to start exercising came while watching the New York City marathon on TV in 1984. Alberto Salazar won it that year. I started running three miles after long work days when I was 36 years old. No previous fitness training. I ran 4-6 days a week, until it caused a strain on my relationship. Training wasn't easy with my strenuous work schedule, but I ran on and off for years. I loved it. I finished my first marathon in 1991 when I was 44 years old. I haven't stopped since.

In my lifetime, I have dealt with hypertension, mild mitral regurgitation (a flow issue in the heart with the mitral valve), anemia, Thyroid Cancer in 2000 (which was cured), and

Degenerative lumbar disk disease. Through it all I still manage to stay competitive in all my races. I always run for time – can't help it! I have to know how I am doing compared to other guys my age.

Before I joined the gym in 2002, the only exercise I ever did was run. But after a shoulder injury from throwing rocks (yes, real rocks), my rehab required exercises like rowing. I saw people doing really active and fun looking exercises in the boxing and bootcamp classes while I forced myself to "row." Exercising should be fun, so I joined in on the classes. Since I had never done anything with weights or tried indoor strength building exercises, they all seemed impossible. I sucked at chin ups, sit ups on the incline board, pushups, jumping rope, wall kicks, gator crawls. But my fitness level has escalated since joining the gym and learning about the other side of being strong. I fell in love with the club boxing classes, and weight training. Where I exercised 4 days a week before the gym, now it's 5 to 6 days a week – both running and the gym.

Exercise has been really positive for me: it changed me from an introvert into an extrovert. I used to be shy, had low self-esteem and even hated myself. Since I started bootcamp, I got hooked on endorphins. I enjoy life, I like people and I even like myself! I have self-confidence.

One of my favorite things about bootcamp: a good instructor, such as Robby. In Robby's class, I enjoy everything, especially: jogging, box jumping, planks (side and regular), sit ups, pushups, jump overs, lunging over the riser the long way (Robby showed me how to do it as a modification to make the station harder). Most of all I enjoy the classmates. The comradery is great and inspiring. I've learned how to talk to other people and everyone is so friendly in class. We all come from different backgrounds but our love of a challenge and of bettering ourselves brings us together. The people are great and so is Robby. I have never seen an instructor put in as much genuine time and care for his class. We even all hang out together outside of class! We go to movies, coffee shops, restaurants. The class has become like family to me.

I try to eat a little healthier (except for the cheat foods) now. I try to get more sleep, and I try to make friends who are active too. The best advice I can share came from a cardiologist who spoke at a wilderness medicine conference in Vale, Colorado. He said, to stay healthy, do whatever exercise you love. As kids, we did what we loved, like riding a bike, playing ball, swimming, etc. If you love the activity, you will never quit. So my advice is that if you attempt something very difficult, like Tabata or P90X, that you don't love, you will soon dread doing it and eventually quit. Do something that you enjoy and you will never stop. I am 68 and getting stronger every day!

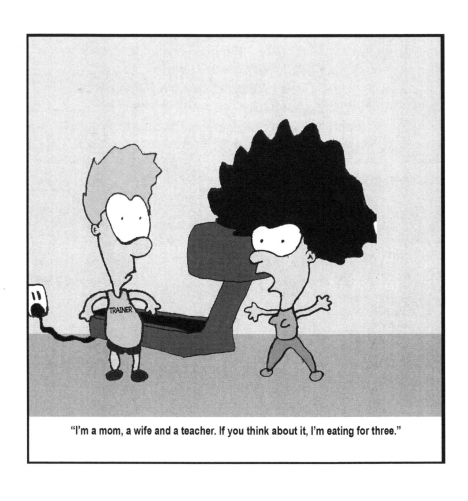

"I'm a mom, a wife and a teacher. If you think about it, I'm eating for three."

"What the mind can conceive, the body can achieve."
- Napoleon Hill

SHANNON

This next woman I'm introducing is a true powerhouse fitness junkie that I've become good friends with. Her name is Shannon and she is a 50-year old woman who is originally from San Diego, California. She claims that her favorite food is anything sweet and of that, her favorite cheat food is donuts. She is currently engaged and so is her fiancé. It hasn't been confirmed but he may have purposed to her by putting her favorite donut around her finger while doing a deep knee lunge. Shannon loves pretty much every exercise except for burpees. Even though she hates doing them, she still does them and I believe one day that it'll be in her top 3 favorite exercises. I'm very happy to have Shannon not only in my class but also as a friend.

Without further adieu, here's Shannon's story:

I was always pretty active as a child and young adult. I played sports and took dance classes, and rode my bike to get places. So as I aged, I didn't really give much thought to staying in shape. As a result, when my activity level dropped off, my weight went up, and my strength and flexibility declined.

At 40 years old I found myself 40-50 pounds overweight, and any exertion was difficult. Like everyone else, I wanted to be thinner, but the thought of what I needed to do was overwhelming. Aside from "the four food groups" I didn't know anything about nutrition, and exercise really didn't sound fun. Besides, I thought, what if I work hard and make sacrifices, and I don't see any results? Everything I read says that moderate exercise for 20 minutes, 3 times a week is all I need to do. So I joined a gym, and randomly went and walked on the treadmill for 20 minutes. Of course, nothing happened, and I quit going. And I didn't change my eating habits. There is so much false information out there: low carb, low fat, high fiber. I didn't really know what to do.

When I got to be around 42 years old, I'd had enough. I knew that anything worth doing was worth doing right. So I joined a gym again, and used my tax refund to hire a trainer for 8 weeks. I was committed. The trainer provided what I really needed: a guarantee that if I did what she said, I would see results. She gave me a meal plan to follow, and I trained with her 3 days a week. At first, I could do very little. I was afraid to do a squat. My balance was so bad that I was afraid I would fall over. Running: are you kidding me? But she encouraged me, and planted the seed in my head that I could do anything I set my mind to. The weight started to drop off. I got stronger. My confidence started to increase. I ran for 30 seconds on the treadmill. Then 45 seconds. Then 60. When I got up to 2 minutes straight I felt like I had achieved an amazing goal! I really could do anything!

I started going to group classes, and making friends at the gym. I enjoyed challenges and competitions. I found that pushing myself gave me a huge sense of accomplishment. And as a side benefit, I could fit into smaller clothes!

When my gym was bought by LA fitness, I wasn't happy. Gone were the trainers that I knew, and the classes that I loved. I was back to feeling a bit lost, and unsure of what I wanted to do at the gym. Running on the treadmill was OK, but not exactly fun.

Then I took Robby's boot camp class. Fun! Positive! A great workout! The social and fun aspect to Robby's teaching style is right up my alley. Bootcamp helped me keep going through the gym transition. It is now the highlight of my week. I'm always sore the next day, but in a good way. The class keeps me motivated to work hard on other days as well. I like that there is always something coming "next" with bootcamp stations. My least favorite exercise, of course, is burpees. But I push through them because I am committed to never let myself get out of shape again.

I did lose the 40 pounds though, happily. That came when I started working out at my first gym 8 years ago. Having Robby's class to look forward to is part of what helps me to keep it off. Mainly, learning to eat right was key. And *wanting* to have good workouts is a constant reminder to eat right.

There is a cycle: eat right to have good workouts, and work out to get the most out of "food fuel."

Life is so much better when you are healthy, and I learned that weight loss isn't the main goal. It's a positive side effect of living a healthy life. And participating in a fun workout that you really connect with helps create and maintain a healthy life.

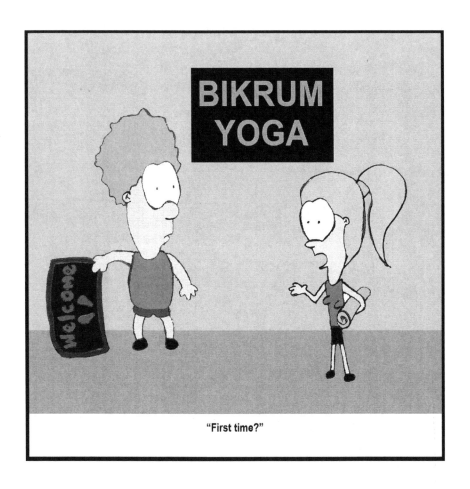

"First time?"

"If you always put limits on everything you do, physical or anything else, it will spread into your work and into your life. There are no limits. There are only plateaus; and you must not stay there, you must go beyond them."

- Bruce Lee

JENNIFER

I'm really pleased to introduce someone who has always been such a good friend to me. Her name is Jennifer and she is 30 plus 5 minus 2 years of age. She is originally from Montrose, Colorado, home of the peaches and now lives in Arizona, home of the peachless. She loves bootcamp in the day and works as an RN at night, which makes her a beast by day and super hero by night. To disguise her powers, she chooses cross-stitching, video games, baking, and crafts as her choice of hobbies. Her favorite cheat food of choice is cheese and wine. Not the fake stuff, either – she'll whine about nacho cheese. Her favorite noise I have not a clue but her favorite class is outdoor bootcamp. I would have to agree with her on that because she told me it was and only she decides what her favorite things are. I'm really happy that she is my friend and the fact that she always expresses how much she appreciates me.
Without further adieu, here's Jennifer's story:

I was always a chubby kid so my parents encouraged me to play sports to lose weight and get healthy. I started with track in middle school and that really helped me to shed my weight. I ended up swimming for my high school. The collage I went to didn't have a swim team so I stopped exercising, gained weight and increased my smoking habit. I knew smoking was damaging to my health on many levels, so I tried to quit on numerous occasions. However, I gained 20 pounds during one of my "quitting" phases, so picked up the habit again to lose the weight. I did, and the smoking also provided me much needed stress relief, albeit temporary.

After moving to Arizona I soon realized that I needed to change my life. I wanted to start with getting healthy again. This time I realized my only way to stay smoke free was to pick up another "habit." The best option I could think of was exercise. Not going to sugarcoat, it was a very painful beginning, but I never gave up. I've been an ex-smoker for over 4 years now!

One of the challenges of exercise for me is that I was born with scoliosis and lordosis of the spine. In high school I developed subluxation of the shoulders and hips (this is basically a temporary dislocation of the joints and can lead to soft tissue damage). There were many exercises along my journey that originally caused pain or that I was simply unable to do. With help from Robby and others with my condition I've learned to modify exercises and increase strength to avoid pain and injury.

Before taking bootcamp I thought that I was in decent shape because of my participation in swimming and cycling classes. After my first bootcamp class, I realized that I was nowhere near the level of fitness I thought I was. The biggest obvious weakness I had was probably not being able to do a single pushup. Holding a one-minute plank was impossible. But I was determined to not give up and push my body to its limits. Probably a full year passed before I became a complete exercise enthusiast. During that time, I came to excel at a one-minute plank. Exercise is a part of my lifestyle now and everything is scheduled around my workout routine. The days that I attend the gym haven't changed: 3-5 depending on my work schedule and other life events. But the duration and intensity of my workouts have increased. Sometimes I go to two fitness classes in one day or do an hour of cardio and an hour of weights. I see the progress my body has made and I feel so good, inside and out.

My favorite part of the bootcamp class is the positive synergism of working out with others who are trying to reach the same goal. Every exercise can be modified and/or substituted, which is great for someone with a chronic condition. Anyone at *any level* can participate and achieve results. Each exercise is done at your own pace, which is extremely appealing when trying something new.

I also still swim, lift weights and attend cycle, boxing and kickboxing classes. Exercise is part of a healthy lifestyle, once you make one healthy choice it's easier to make another. Eventually most of your choices will be healthy and positive with fewer and fewer bad choices polluting your life.

Exercise is the ultimate stress reliever. Sometimes my job is very demanding and can take a toll physically and spiritually. When I attend bootcamp my focus is on what my body is doing and stretching its limits. Afterwards, the endorphins are overflowing and the stress of both work and life melt away. That is why it is worth it to me to keep up my weekly workout schedule.

Whatever exercise you choose to do, make sure you enjoy it and look forward to participating the next time. If you have to force yourself to do something, odds are you won't do it for very long and you will give up. If you've never exercised before, try it for 15 minutes, then 30, then 60. The all or nothing attitude should not be a part of a healthy lifestyle. It's ok to indulge every now and again. Never follow fad diets or restrict your diet to the point of being miserable. In the end, it's your life and you should live it how you want to without restraint. Positive results will lead you to make more positive choices. I can't imagine my life without fitness now. Taking care of and challenging my body are a part of who I am, a part I am extremely proud of.

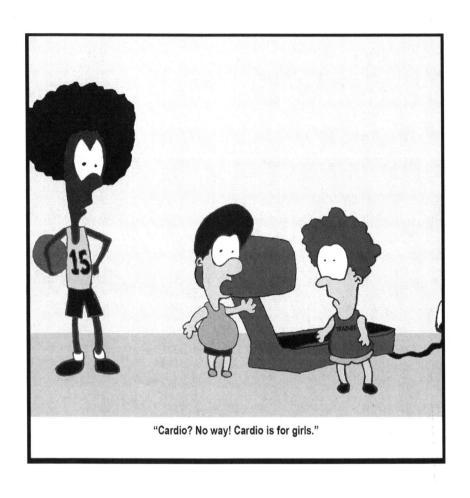

"Health is not valued until sickness comes."
- Thomas Fuller

MAUREEN

I'm very happy to introduce this next woman who I consider a sweet friend of mine. Her name is Maureen and she is a 58-year old woman from Johnstown, Pennsylvania. She is recently married and between her husband and herself, they share 4 daughters, 3 son-in-law's, 5 grandchildren, and hundreds of bags of Dorito's chips. She loves snicker doodle cookies because of the name and taste...but mainly the name. When she's not traveling the world, she spends her free time volunteering or working out. Besides bootcamp, some of her workouts include: hiking, hot yoga, walking, and diving – which in my imagination, is her diving from 1,500 feet up and doing dozens of flips in the process. I'd ask her to elaborate but I'm happy with my own story of her diving adventures and that is what I tell people. Maureen is as sweet as she is strong and I am happy that she takes my class and is someone that I can call my friend.
Without further adieu, here's Maureen's story:

I've been an exercise enthusiast/advocate for as long as I can remember. From the time I was 20, there hasn't been a time I haven't been active: biking, taking ballet, taking classes at gyms, etc. Even when I was busy having babies, I worked out at home to exercise tapes. I've always loved that I not only see improvement in my strength, tone, endurance and flexibility, but I also make friends. The friends I have made in my classes are not only fun to be around, but they also keep me accountable. It's not unusual to hear, "will you be here tomorrow?" I look forward to seeing my gym friends and family.

When I started taking bootcamp with Robby, I was unsure. It just sounded so difficult and intimidating. However, this class is the best! The different stations include physical training, cardio, core and toning. During class, Robby constantly moves from station to station, where he gives tips, checks alignment, is cognizant of your strengths and weaknesses and will adjust a segment if you have an injury. He gives us attention and knows his students as if he were your own personal trainer. In the beginning, I really didn't care for burpees. They were so hard. I felt like they were way too hard for "an old lady," but now when I hear them called for at one of the stations, I don't even blink an eye. I feel stronger now and can do them correctly and efficiently. I feel burpees are a vital part of the total body workout in bootcamp.

My weekly workouts usually include 1-2 full body sessions, step class, hot yoga, walking and of course, bootcamp. I feel as though I am taking care of myself through these classes, relieving stress and keeping my attitude positive. This attitude follows me from the gym, where it affects decisions regarding nutrition, family dynamics, and my relationships. I feel blessed that I have the time and ability to work out frequently and plan to continue this lifestyle as long as I possibly can.

I appreciate instructors like Robby who keep me motivated, safe, and who have a genuine interest in my health and well-being. I am glad I took a chance on bootcamp. I always look forward to this class. Robby also injects his wit and personal stories into class. By doing this, he is more "human," approachable, and one of us. I feel Robby regards us not only as his students but as his friends!

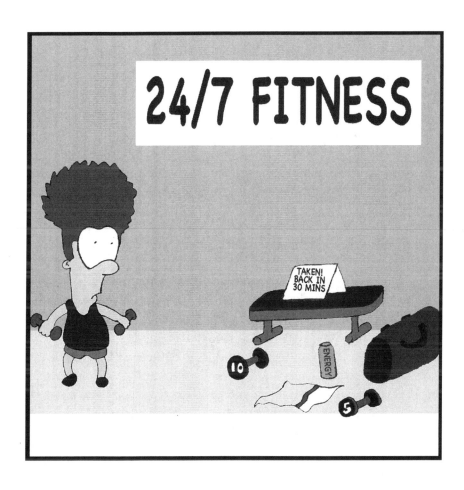

"Fresh air impoverishes the doctor."
- Danish Proverb

KENDRA

It's my pleasure to introduce this next person that I call friend. Her name is Kendra and she is one of the most positive people I know, even in times of high stress. I think her secret super power is her ability to have fun with others. She has a natural ability to bring out the fun in others and that's just one of the reasons why people cling to her. When she isn't traveling all over the country, she spends 1/3 of her time in the gym and 2/3 of her time outdoors climbing on things – mostly rocks, mountains, and trees. I appreciate her friendship and the love she spreads to everyone in she comes in contact with. It's a quality everyone should adopt and continuously practice each day.

Without further adieu, here's Kendra's story:

My name is Kendra and I am 31 years old, married three happy years. I think everyone needs a good dose of Vitamin D, which, translated means I love to be outdoors as much as possible. I have been known to integrate yoga into several outdoor activities, whether it be hiking or paddle boarding. I also really love my mud runs. Everything I do, I like to do with others. I love helping people get healthy, which has led me into a nursing career. I have been in the healthcare industry 12 years, serving as a nurse for the last 2.

I grew up in Colorado so being active outdoors was always easy. In junior high I played soccer and then in high school I ran cross country. Later on I snowboarded, rode bikes a lot, roller-bladed, and hiked. I just loved being outside! When I moved to Arizona 7 years ago staying active with these hobbies became a lot more challenging so I joined a gym. I've always done group fitness there. It's rare that I will go to the gym and work out by myself. If my husband joins me, we will do a floor workout. Otherwise, I am in classes 4-6 times a week.

There was a brief period during nursing school when I gained weight and didn't work out as much as I used to. I got too heavy and out of shape to feel good anymore. This was my "woah" moment. Everyone needs a "woah" moment. I knew something had to change. It was during this time that I met Robby and started taking his bootcamp class at the gym. I started going back to classes more and got off the steak and pizza diet. I started eating more protein and being more conscious about what I ate. I have been able to lose the nursing school weight and I feel so much better. I sleep better. When good nutrition gets added to your life, the difference in how you feel is amazing. A combo of exercise and good nutrition makes for such a more energetic and happy life.

I usually rotate between three different classes; cycle, weights, and bootcamp. Bootcamp really pushes me. I like the socializing that comes with the workout. I feel like taking bootcamp regularly keeps me fit. In the beginning it was definitely a challenge, just like anything new. Tricep dips were hard to keep up for the allotted time in the beginning. Getting over the mindset, "I gotta do it for two minutes?!" was tough. But in fitness, it doesn't get easier: you just get better. Now I rock out triceps, but burpees are still really challenging for me. I don't love them, but what doesn't challenge you doesn't change you.

You have to want positive change in your life, or it won't stick. I love my healthy, active lifestyle. I would never want to live any other way. I still have my "cheat" moments. I still love pizza and steak now and then, and I love Mexican food. Honestly, I just love food in general! But I don't believe in diets. The word "diet" suggests something that is not sustainable. I believe in following a fit lifestyle that can work for everyone, for life.

I can't even imagine – nor would I want to- life without bootcamp classes and other fun physical activities.

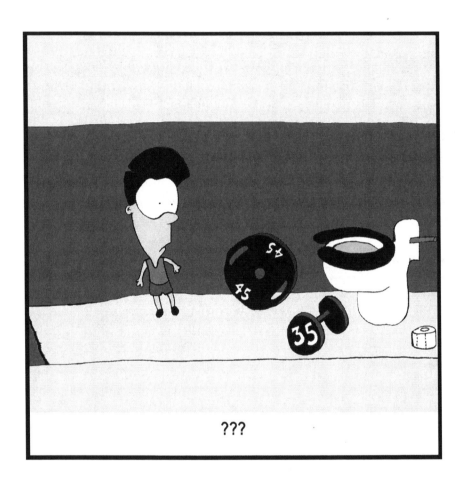

"Take care of your body. It's the only place you have to live."
- Jim Rohn

IZAMAR

The first time I met Izamar, I thought she had made up her name when I asked her what it was. But, I didn't question it and it turned out she was telling me the truth. I knew that from the moment I saw her friend request on Facebook- this was no fake profile. I see that she goes by "Isa" and I'll tell you now that she definitely "is a" training beast in a small package. She's a 22-year old Hispanic woman from Santana, California who loves enchiladas. I was curious what her favorite cheat food was and completely surprised to know it was Wendy's. I don't know if she dips her fries in their frostys or not but I do know that I would if I still ate there....but I don't. She enjoys writing and learning new things, as well as going on hikes and being out in nature. She shares some of my favorite exercises, which are squats and lunges and I think that "is a" very awesome thing!
Without further adieu, here's Izamar's story:

My name is Izamar Martinez (Izzy) I am a 23-year old female who wasn't always fond of exercising. A few years ago I was not even considering exercising or anything which involved my health. Three years of procrastination - yes three – had kept me out of the gym. Then one day I realized I come from a long line of cardiac and diabetes health problems. As I was sitting down at the bus stop staring at a tall building backed by huge mountains, I saw a metaphor of all my life obstacles, those past and those I will face in the future.

I said to myself, "Enough Izzy! Take control stop being afraid!"

A huge flaw of mine is not taking the necessary risks which later on will benefit me.

I was 21 when I decided to enroll at a gym and take the time to start a healthy lifestyle. As I sat down with a sales rep and went through the process of learning more about the facility I couldn't believe myself. I, Izamar Martinez was signing a way to a new, fresh start! I was introduced to the head trainer of the facility and booked a free, one-time session. He asked me why I joined. *Why*, a question which I had only one answer to:

"I want to start a new, healthy lifestyle. I want to feel better about myself."

When family and friends found out I joined the gym and had a personal trainer I did not always get a positive reaction.

"Why did you join the gym, you are already skinny?" Or,

"You will look like a stick when you are done."

My first training session was awful. I felt as if I was going to die. I honestly wanted to quit, I didn't feel strong like I now feel. It was the hardest thing I have ever experienced. I had to stand in front of a mirror and start a pep talk before every training session. I went to the gym three to four times a week: it was a way to cope with stress from work and school. My first trainer was so motivating and other trainers high-fived me whenever I accomplished a task. One trainer always gave me hope: Austin constantly made me feel better about myself by giving me so much praise. My self-esteem increased drastically.

One day I said, "SCREW THIS! I am doing this for me and my health and not to impress anyone!"

It took me three years and seven months to acknowledge how strong I am mentally and physically. I found a motivation to keep me going on all the workout plans my new trainer Arthur had planned for me. That motivation was my education. I finally realized *why* God has me on this Earth: I am here to help others. So I applied for the bilingual nursing program at the college I attended. Unfortunately, I haven't been accepted yet. It is the hardest program to be admitted to but I will not stop. When I am in the middle of lifting weights or running I keep my focus on my degree and future patients I will soon be helping with a smile across my face. When I finish the workout plan my trainer has set up for me I feel as if I have accomplished my future. I will make a difference in their lives and make a change to those in third world countries. As Ghandi said, "Be the change you wish to see in the world."

A year ago I attended Robby's bootcamp class. My coworker finally convinced me to go with her. It was intense but worth it. He came around and made sure I was doing the exercise correct so I wouldn't hurt myself. Being in Robby's class was the first time I have ever felt accepted by anyone: I wasn't judged by how I look or my spunky personality. Honestly, I felt as if I was home. I had fun and couldn't wait to go again.

There were days where I wasn't able to attend during the week due to my class schedule but I would go in on Saturdays or Sundays. I even attended a 5k run with the bootcamp class. I didn't run the whole thing: sometimes I walked when I started to feel tired, but I did not quit. I kept my focus on nursing and ended the race.

Unfortunately, it has now been seven months since I have set foot in the gym. I injured myself; tore my meniscus while doing suicides (running drills). I had surgery on July 2 and am not yet done with therapy. I will soon get back to the gym. I have to take it easy at first, of course; baby steps. The rehab will all be worth it. I can't wait to get back to class and to pushing myself again.

Remember: do things you want for yourself only. In the end, this life and how you spend your time is all about your health and happiness.

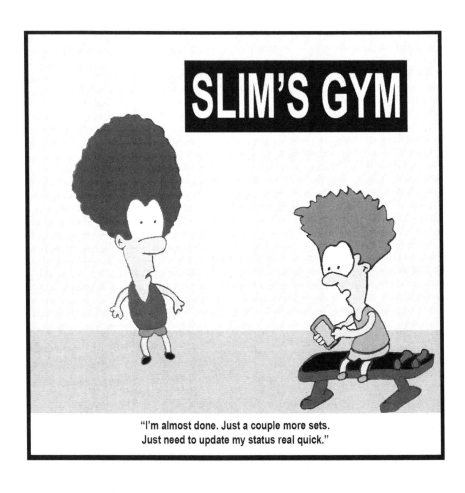

"The more you're obsessed by something, believing it, the better chance you have of achieving it."

- Frank Zane

VICTOR

This next guy I'm introducing is 58 years old, Hispanic and a retired Mesa Municipal Court judge. That's right! He's single with two grown kids and one of the nicest people you'll ever meet. He enjoys camping, hunting, fishing, and his favorite food is salmon. He likes to treat himself, every now and then, on tamales. I remember Victor's first class. I see him in class today and can see a big difference in his energy, endurance, and strength. When I stopped teaching at the original club where he would attend, I wanted to stay in touch with him. He mentioned he had a Facebook account and it took about a month because he didn't have a profile picture up (and I don't add anyone without that at least). A mutual friend connected with him and taught him how to upload a photo. He had just one photo and finally, after about a year, he now has two. I'm very happy to be friends with Victor and I'm even happier that he trusts my instruction and takes my classes. It means a lot to me that a man like him saw good judgment in me.
Without further adieu, here's Victor's story:

I have been weight lifting and playing basketball since high school. Like so many avid basketball players, eventually I had to have knee surgery. I began taking bootcamp about 6 months after my surgery and stuck with it throughout my rehab. I was limited at some stations but my condition never stopped me from getting sweaty and pushing myself to grow healthier. I have had to give up basketball since my surgery. I miss the competitiveness and fast pace of the game. But bootcamp has given me something new and challenging to look forward to.

After just one month of bootcamp, I was hooked. I had worked out 4-5 days a week before I started bootcamp, but I was doing the same routine and exercises so was in a rut. Burpees and pushups were hard for all 6'2", 240 pounds of me, but now I can finish the sets at each station and push out a solid performance in the group challenge as well.

I thought I was in decent shape before I started bootcamp

since I had stayed active with basketball all my life. But I have since seen so much progression. Even with the setback in my knee, my strength and endurance have grown tremendously. I feel so much better. My stress levels have also lowered. The group setup of bootcamp make it so that I am working out around other athletes. Some are advanced and I strive to reach their level. Some of these competitors are female, some are older males, some are different ethnicities, and almost all are different body types. But I have a competitive side that is drawn to the never ending challenge of class.

Every area of my life is better after becoming part of the bootcamp family. I eat better at home. I feel better all the time. My knee is gaining mobility and strength. I am able to destress after a long week of working (I went back as a judge for the family courts, part time because I didn't like the slow pace of retirement.)

Don't be afraid to make a change when life throws you a challenge. I hated giving up basketball. It was a part of my life for so long. Even though I love bootcamp, of course I still miss the unique aspects of the game. But I am commited to taking care of my body as I age and basketball threatens my mobility now. So I have taken a turn in my life journey. I have become a bootcamp junkie. I have made new friends who notice when I am not in class. I have made new goals and pushed my body toward achieving them. Making new friends to inspire me have been a powerful plus.

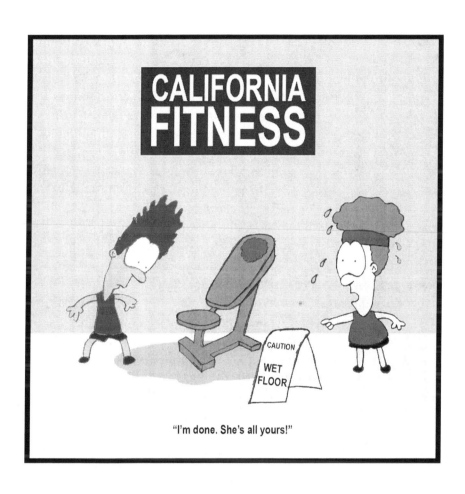

"Exercise is so amazing from the inside out. I feel so alive and have so much energy."

- Vanessa Hudgens

CLARE

I'm very pleased to introduce you to this next woman. Her name is Clare and she is a 50-year old Psychologist from Dillon, Montana – a large city with more than 4,000 residents. She's single with no kids but has a big interest in genealogy. Like me, some of her favorite cheat foods are scones with cream and Trader Joe's Mini Dark Chocolate bars. Even though she lives in Phoenix, Arizona and has access to many indoor local gyms, Clare still enjoys nature's gym of being outside. Her favorite exercise is hiking the mountains in Montana. If it were possible, she would fly out there each day before work to hike. And although she gives a lot of credit to many of the people and instructors in her life for her amazing progress in fitness, it's my opinion that she is just one of the stronger people who have real self-motivation for more strength and a desire to grow. She's not just an intelligent person who wanted change, she's a person who chose a plan of action and saw it through by putting in her own hard work and determination. I'm very happy that she decided to share her story because I know that many people will connect with her and the journey she's on. Thank you for your friendship and for being a part of the fitness family we all have in each other.

Without further adieu, here's Clare's story:

Growing up on a farm in rural Montana, I spent the majority of my time outdoors. We could walk for miles behind our house and never run into another person. Together with my five younger sisters, we constantly ran up hills, swam in freezing lakes and coasted our bikes down the steep mountain pass near our home.

In contrast, now I live in Central Phoenix and spend much of my life in an office. While in my 20s and still in grad school, I made a commitment to exercise in order to maintain my health. I had been diagnosed with hypothyroid and, ultimately, this called my attention to the importance of staying in shape. It seemed strange to exercise in a gym after all those years of running through the fields of southwest Montana and, in truth, I still find it odd. However, I decided that my sedentary career demanded I join the urban ritual of gym membership. After all, I couldn't realistically spend my days moving irrigation pipe and chasing down wayward sheep.

For many years, I worked out in a gym on my own or with a few friends. It took me a long time to garner the courage to participate in group classes. As a PE flunky, I was traumatized at the mere thought of group work-outs. I was afraid of looking like a fool – this comes from a person who on one occasion almost shot the gym teacher with an arrow!

About five years ago, I realized that I needed to step up my exercise routine because I wasn't getting results on my own. I was mid-way through my 40s and dealing with complications from hypothyroid that resulted in *dragging* through work-outs. As I lifted free weights, I observed several classes through the glass and realized that I could probably handle them without too much humiliation. I started going to BodyWorks classes (weights) and eventually incorporated spin into my routine. I have terribly flat feet and zero rhythm so I gave up on Zumba after one class.

For quite some time, I observed the energy and camaraderie of Robby's bootcamp as I waited for the class immediately after. I was intimidated by bootcamp but noticed that quite a few elderly women participated and everyone seemed to have a good time! I decided to give it a try and am now a convert! I love Robby's bootcamp because of the great energy and supportive participants. Robby is kind and welcoming to everyone, regardless of their fitness level. He creates an environment where everyone belongs.

I take my gym commitments seriously and if I don't exercise for a few days, I get cranky. Exercise helps keep me sane in a challenging job and is a major stress outlet. Because of the various classes I attend, I have built core strength. A few years ago, I started experiencing lower back pain, probably due to sitting so much during the day. I no longer experience any discomfort and owe it all to fitness instructors who got me into shape.

Although I've always eaten fairly healthy foods, I have eliminated almost all sugar from my diet and am working toward being gluten-free. Exercise and nutrition go hand-in-hand and each one reinforces the other. Being in shape makes me want to eat better!

This year I turned 50 and can honestly say that I am in better shape than I was in my 20s and 30s. Although I will never be much of an athlete, I feel really good about my fitness level. The ongoing issues with hypothyroid and a genetic predisposition put me at high risk for osteoporosis, but recently I underwent a bone density scan and the results were above average for my age group! All the hard work pays off! I am very aware that I'm not working out solely for the present moment but also in hopes to remain healthy throughout the entire course of my life. My personal goals are these: to complete 20 perfect burpees in a row and never spend a single night in a hospital.

I know one thing for certain: I could never have done this on my own. I am immensely grateful to dedicated teachers like Robby who are encouraging and welcoming and who help us become more fit than we ever imagined! Thank you for helping me age with grace, strength and health.

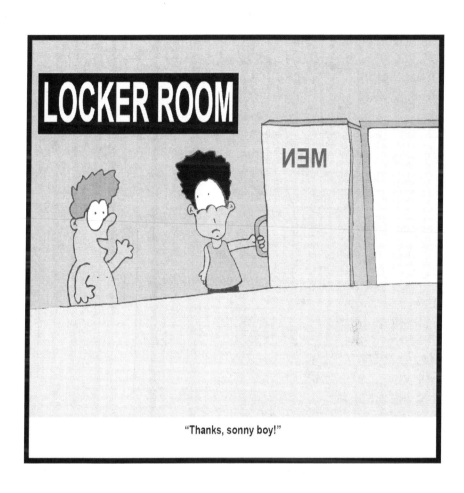

"A man too busy to take care of his health is like a mechanic too busy to take care of his tools."

- Spanish Proverb

RODOLFO

I'm very pleased to introduce this next guy who I call my friend. His name is Rodolfo and he is single guy who makes time for his workouts even though he is busy with several jobs. It's been a pleasure to see his hard work pay off in class and I'm honored that he gives me credit even though it was off his own hard work and dedication. Rodolfo snapped a quick selfie of us at the last class he was at and posted it up on Facebook. To this day, we can't get any peace with the hundreds of modeling and acting agencies begging us to star in upcoming films. They think we're playing hard to get but really, we're just busy killing it in the gym, which is our main priority. Thank you for your friendship and for being part of this book!

Without further adieu, here's Rodolfo's story:

My name is Rodolfo Gomez. I am a 30-year old single male. I was born in Mexico and came to the United States 14 years ago. I work in both construction and the restaurant industry. When not working hard I enjoy hiking, and bike riding. My favorite food is sushi. I like to go out to Kona Grill with friends. When I am not caring about eating healthy I love Vaqueros Mexican food.

I have always been a big man. If you saw me a year ago, you would not even recognize me. I have been taking bootcamp classes for 1 year and 2 months. Because of the challenging and positive class, and with Robby's help, I have been able to lose 50 pounds! I feel energy all day long and I'm filled with a strength that I get from class. But in the beginning, everything was really hard for me. I wasn't even able to run for more than five minutes. If there were levels to running, I was on level -3!

I started out exercising only two days a week at the gym. First I lifted weights, and then I went into bootcamp. When I lost most of my weight I was working out five times a week. My first bootcamp class was hard! I wanted to throw up, actually. But I really liked the trainer. Robby is very motivating. By far the hardest exercise I did was suicides.

Now that I have lost 50 pounds and gained strength, I want to maintain, and I just workout whenever I can. My favorite part of bootcamp is pushups. While I used to be a "-3" runner, now I can go to Tempe Town Lake a jog for 45 minutes. I work harder in classes now and I can work two jobs, no problemo. Also I feel confident with myself: I have more respect for myself and for my body. I can pull up my shirt without feeling bad! (Ok, I'm still feeling shy but not nearly as embarrassed as before.) I love challenging myself. I enjoy challenging myself with all the other people in class. Everyone is doing the same activities that I like, and we are all making gains and feeling satisfied together.

If I could share anything with others who want to make a big change in their lives, I would say to them, "You're gonna be healthy! People are gonna look at you differently and you are going to feel amazing! Your self-esteem will go up if you exercise. You will wake up in the mornings with a positive mind: exercise and healthy eating changes the way you think and live your life."

I still have a long way to go. More weight to lose and more strength to gain. But today, I feel really good. I am so happy that I met Robby and have had his classes to support me in my weight loss.

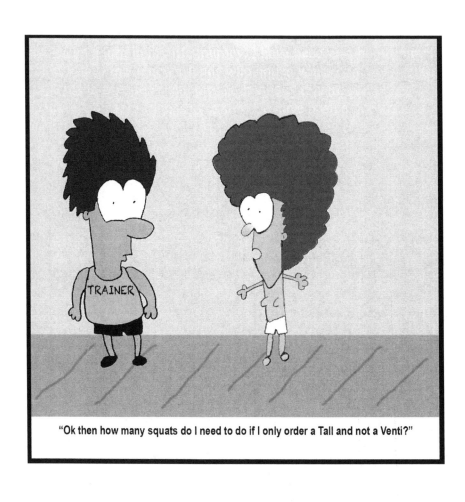

"Ok then how many squats do I need to do if I only order a Tall and not a Venti?"

"The best doctor gives the least medicines."
- Benjamin Franklin

BRIAN

It's with great pleasure I introduce my friend, Brian. Being half Irish and half French, Brian chose teaching high school Spanish as his career choice. Since the early '60's, he fell in love with the culture and to this day, visits Mexico on business trips and to see good friends about 5 times per year. He keeps the culture alive in Phoenix by eating at some of the best authentic restaurants in town. I first met Brian a couple years ago when he attended a class I subbed at the gym and am happy to see him still attending regularly each week. Being that he's 70 years old and still coming to class full of energy and good spirits, I feel he's an inspiration to many who are around him. I asked what his favorite exercise was and he immediately blurted out in Spanish "push-ups" and dropped and gave me twenty as he counted in Spanglish. He has two grown kids, spends his free time reading and continuing education, works out regularly, and eats Santa Fe Burgers and Cajun fries to splurge. He is living a very fulfilled and purposeful life and brings smiles to everyone he's in contact with. Many can learn from this man and I'm very proud to call him my friend.

Without further adieu, here's Brian's story:

As a 16-year old, I wanted to be muscular so I would look sexy. Thus began my fitness career. As I matured, the high I experienced after a workout along with the energy and health benefits kept me exercising. I lifted weights in my house in my early days of exercising, but running has always been my favorite way to stay in shape. In 1980, at age, 45, I joined a gym. It was giant old, rickety bikes and utilitarian machines in those days. Group classes looked more like dance videos and I stayed away from them.

Two years ago, when I first walked into a boot camp class on a Sunday morning, the most difficult parts of the hour were the cardio--running and skipping. I was 68 years old and working on my wind, but progress was – and still is – slow. Soon Robby took over the bootcamp class and I loved it just as much as before. I have had to cut back drastically on my outdoor running now that I am in my 70s, and Robby's class helps me keep up my lung strength.

I work out five to six days a week: take bootcamp on two of those days. I also do Robby's cycle class and one weights class a week. Regardless of some of the difficulties that could discourage me, there is no better feeling than the exhilarated, "pumped" feeling I have after class. I even have that feeling the days I walk out of class tired. And I sleep well at night because of the frequent exercise. I also don't mind keeping the same pant size year after year.

Good and not so good instructors come and go. Robby is certainly among the good that you hope will never leave. Because of his gentle yet energetic spirit, Robby's classes have been a great motivator in my quest to stay fit and energetic myself for as long as I can. The routines he sets out for us are always challenging but with attainable goals that keep me trying. I love the variety in bootcamp stations. The only time I feel my age is when I have to walk or slow down. But I have learned to listen to my body and find a balance between exertion and rest. If I need to walk during a jog warm up one day, I do it with a smile. And it really doesn't matter – everyone in class is on their own level. I always hear positive feedback from people around me.

Robby's bootcamp – and I underscore "Robby's," has turned into a community. It's great to encourage others and be encouraged by them. Getting to know the people in class with me every week has been so interesting. We carry on our friendships outside of class. Robby will often stop to visit during an exercise; just today he was explaining to me how little weight you need to exercise the shoulder rotators to keep them in shape.

I know many of us felt the loss and the vacuum when he decided not to teach Sunday mornings. On the other hand, I'm glad that he knew what was good for himself. I look forward to every Thursday, my only class with Robby now: it is an integral part of my week. I'm never sluggish after bootcamp. I may have some muscular pain, but that just tells me I am doing something right. I always associate muscular pain with getting stronger.

Some of the younger people in class tell me I am an inspiration to them. I hope I can be. My commitment to fitness and my health is a big part of what keeps me happy. We can't stop time, but we can savor it.

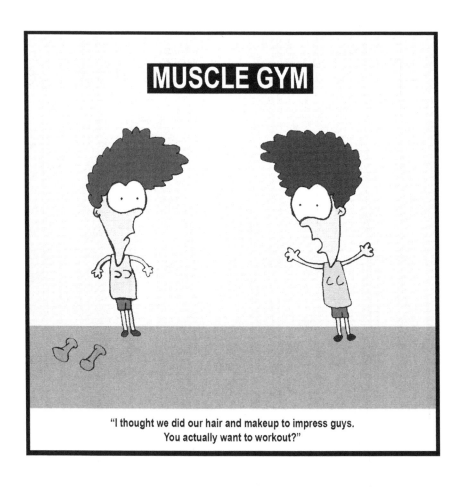

"In the confrontation between the stream and the rock, the stream always wins. Not through strength, but through persistence."

- H. Jackson Brown, Jr.

VIRGIL

It's an honor for me to introduce this next friend of mine. His name is Virgil and he really is a one-of-a-kind friend in my life. Although he has a couple years on me, we share many similarities and had we gone to the same school growing up, we probably would've been really close friends. Many people miss him as he travels all over the U.S. – usually leaving without telling anyone ahead of time but he makes sure to tag everyone in the photos he takes at all the cool places he visits. He's probably the biggest 49ers fan there is and they should put him on payroll for all the marketing he's done for them. I'm very happy to have him as my friend and any one of his friends would tell you the same. Thank you for being a part of this book and thank you more for always being such a great friend to me.

Without further adieu, here's Virgil's story:

I am 49 years old and I've been into fitness since I started elementary school. I love being active and having fun with it. I was in sports in Jr high and high school: cross country, football, basketball and track. I think it was because of my passion for sports that I had the eye for the military. I knew the army would help keep me fit and get stronger. I felt most at home when I was active. I served in the United States Army for 5 years.

Unfortunately, something besides the military was also a big part of my life: drinking. I drank heavily during my time serving all over the world. I missed out on enjoying sights and cultures of the world because I was drinking so much while off duty. I kept at it after I got out and it hindered my fitness. On a Monday I would say, "man, I gotta work out." I'd work out 2-3 days and go back into drinking as the weekend approached. You just can't mix the two together.

The guys that really inspired me to get into running back in the '80s and be strong were Bill Rogers, Steve Ovett, Sebastian Coe, and Alberto Salazar. I followed them and wanted to be like them. But my party life held me back.

My drinking continued to take over and really grew out of hand. It started to affect family and me as a person. I wasn't able to be consistent with anything. I was angry all the time; a nice guy during the week but a monster over the weekends. I was in and out of jail for fights and other stupid arrests dealing with alcohol.

About five years ago I really wanted a change. I knew I had to quit drinking. I went to church, sometimes with a hangover. I sat in the back row next to a guy named Harold. We didn't say much, but always sat next to one another in the back row. One day, I talked to my pastor about my struggles to kick the habit. He referred me to a recovering alcoholic. He said I might know him, because I sat next to him every week in church. It was Harold. I still get chills when I share the story. Harold had two years of sobriety and he took me to AA meetings and served as my mentor. It was fate. I went to AA 20-30 times; usually the Indian AA meetings on Friday nights at 8:00. That was my new happy hour.

They asked people to donate at the end of each meeting. Every week the pot was full of court ordered probation sheets (60 plus), needing a signature proving that their owner's attended. I was one of maybe 7 people who were there voluntarily. I didn't stay too long in AA because I knew what my weakness was and really wanted the change. I knew what I had to do to stay away from alcohol.

I decided to join a gym during that time. My main goal when I first started was to attend group boxing classes. Even now, I shoot for the gym so I can educate myself and then help other Natives get fit. The stereotype is that all Natives are out-of-shape alcoholics. Let's change that. I wanted to be strong and healthy and help mentor Natives into this happier, stronger lifestyle.

I was taking classes regularly when Robby started teaching. This was over two years ago. The gym was doing away with boxing classes and replacing them with Zumba. Robby came just in time to save me from that craziness. He started up a bootcamp. I tried his class and said right away, "Man, this guy's good." Robby locked me in. I ended up travelling really far 4 times a week just to go to his class because he was so motivating. I loved the comradery there. The way he has everything set up is really cool and the "Bubble Gum" music gets me pumped up. Trying to raise those legs up with wall kicks was the hardest thing for me! I still can't get them up high enough, geez! But I can do solid military pushups and deep squats. My cardio got a lot better too, taking his class.

His outdoor bootcamp set up especially reminds me of the military. Certain exercises and the style of carrying them out reflects back on that type of motivation that I received in the Army. I love it.

Staying fit keeps me disciplined. I get complimented at work for my hard work ethic, for not quitting and not whining. I also notice that I am not tired all the time now that I workout several times a week. The new type of friends that I have made at the gym are the type who want to better themselves instead of party. Everyone, I mean, everyone there has beautiful stories. We inspire each other and learn from one another. We keep each other coming back each week. I feel like the gym people are family.

I have made up my mind that I will never drink again. Even when work takes me out of state and away from gyms, I don't go back to the bottle. Being sober has really enabled me to stay fit, be healthier and consistently be who I want to be. I also stay fit because I want to beat the odds. Being Native, I know I have many health risks. There are so many Natives who, when they drink, go extreme. Many end up with diabetes. I want to keep away from all of that and help other Natives be healthy and successful in the process.

Nutrition is what I need to learn more about and focus more on now. If I can pair that with my workouts I know I will get even stronger, not get injured, and be able to be successful in any goal I make. Anyone thinking about making a change in their life, getting healthy, I say, just do it. I still get as much of a high in Robby's class as I did in the beginning. I do 5k runs when I am out of town. I've even been known to hit the deck in a hotel room to "push 'em out," knowing that my bootcamp friends back home expect no less from me. And I still got a lot more left in this journey of mine.

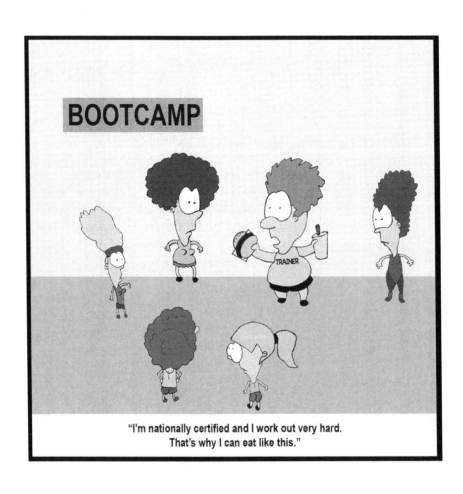

"I'm not a health freak. I just work out every day."
- Anthony Hopkins

KELLY

This next friend of mine is one of the most amazing people I know and over the last year, she has become one of my closest friends. Her name is Kelly and she is an extraordinarily pretty 36-year old red headed super mom of 4 children, real estate agent, fitness freak, hair stylist, and lover of the great outdoors who lives in Chandler, Arizona. She is also known globally for her quick wit and amazing sense of humor. Also, a fun fact about Kelly is that she will fight just about anyone if chocolate is on the line. I remember her first bootcamp class was actually a trap set up with a chocolate trail on the ground that lead from her car to inside the classroom...and the chocolate wasn't even wrapped. There are many wonderful things that I could say that couldn't possibly describe her in full. But, I will say that she's always been attentive in my life and has always lifted me up when I've been down. I'm very grateful for our friendship and for someone who truly cares about me. Not only is she a bright spot in my life; she lights up the world up without even trying. Thank you for being a part of this book, the world is lucky to have someone like you bringing happiness to so many.

Without further adieu, here's Kelly's story:

Misery and betrayal snapped me awake into a life that reflected other people's dreams rather than my own. At once I knew I would *never... ever...* get back so many wasted years. And if I didn't start living outwardly who I was on the inside, too soon there might literally not be any life left.

I was 33; a mother of four. My youngest was only a few months old and still nursing. I needed to connect with life again; if not for my sake then for theirs. I felt trapped, literally and emotionally on a tiny island off the Puget Sound. One morning I wiped away tears and pulled out a notebook, writing across the top of a blank page, "What would make me happy?"

"Fitness: being strong/healthy," wrote out a meager voice inside that still sparked.

As a child I saw Linda Hamilton physically transform

herself in Terminator 2, working her upturned steel bed frame as a pull up bar in a sparse cell. This brief image left a profound mark. Never had I seen such proactive transformation in a woman. I longed to be strong like her, though without any examples or direction. All these years later, the appeal of feminine strength still moved me.

I determined to exercise three set days a week. I treated this new "me time" like a job. I downloaded a free Couch Potato to 5K app and bought a used double stroller with a rain cover to house my two-year old and his baby sister. No excuses. I obediently jogged and walked in rain or winds all over my island, stopping too many times to count for a crying baby or hungry toddler. Then I joined a free boot camp-style fitness group that met in a friend's home twice a week. Sometimes dishes went undone, or a meeting was missed, but the satisfaction I felt from each small fitness gain kept me faithful to my regimen. My spirit healed and grew as my body went from being able to run a few minutes at a time to a half hour. The first time I did 12 burpees in a row left me glowing all week. *Watch out, Linda Hamilton, I'm comin' for ya!*

I lost 10 lbs of baby weight and grew muscle I didn't even know I had during that first year of bringing Kelly back. I couldn't sleep the night before my first adult 5k. I showed up, ran hard into powerful ocean headwinds, and got beat out by an old man. He did have exceptionally long, gangly marathoner legs... What a rush to participate though! Not just daydream, but DO! I was hooked on fitness.

Then an abrupt move from my small island town back to the big desert city threatened to derail my efforts. But since exercise had been a huge part of saving my life, I had to find a way to honor it. For the first time in 15 years, I joined a gym. I felt alien on the gym floor, but hoped to find a class with the challenge and friendships like I had gained on the island. I kept my morning schedule and showed up, alone and shy, to my first gym bootcamp. The music was charged and the energy was catching. Robby's leadership style made me feel both at ease and also driven to work hard. I laughed out loud at the insanity of him expecting us to do wall kicks for two minutes straight. And forget 12 burpees- he expected us to do them nonstop for a minute! But I wasn't the only one who had to laugh away the sweat and go home sore. I loved both my bootcamp and weights classes and soon progressed from three days a week to six. Each small gain at the gym filled me with such satisfaction and excitement. No day was complete without sweat. Exercise was finally the priority in my life that I had always fantasized about.

In the beginning, I could count on Robby's bootcamp to stick to my sore muscles for two days. A year later, I may happily take a little soreness home now and then, but not without adding some solo gym floor time to each bootcamp workout. I love that while now wall kicks are the easy part of class I am still challenged with a fun, full-body workout. There is always a new goal to work towards. The music still pumps me up. Now I work out beside friends of all ages and backgrounds. These friends I cherish because they see an unfiltered me and actually like her! We all go home to differing lives, but are joined in bootcamp by our love and need for fitness. My spark of self and of confidence has spread into a fire.

I did lose a few things going to bootcamp: unwanted weight and a taste for crap foods. As I grew stronger not only did I lose weight but my body craved higher quality foods. I can no longer stomach much of the junk that once was a normal part of my diet. Better nutrition benefits my body, my mind, my emotions and certainly my family. The only part of me that has fattened up is my patience, which was slim before. Surpassing so many goals has taught me that I can achieve anything with daily effort and time.

Giving myself permission to value my health was the most direct step I have ever taken toward happiness. It's been amazing to see and feel the transformation. I used to think "fit" people were just different than me. But now I know we are what we do, and coupling time with effort makes anything possible. A few months ago a woman in class grasped my arms and exclaimed, "Honey, what are you doing here? If I had a body like yours I wouldn't come to class!"

I smiled knowingly: *I wouldn't have this body if I didn't come to class.*

We may not control the genetic earth from which our bodies' spring, but we can choose how to shape and tone our landscape. We only get one life and one body, and happiness cannot truly be enjoyed in the one without care for the other. As you grow physically stronger, new energy will flow over into other parts of your life. Like a drop of water rippling outward, becoming an ocean of waves, your health is more powerful and far reaching that you can even imagine. I feel happier now than I ever have. Last month I was too busy mastering pull ups with amazing people to make lists about what might bring future happiness.

Bootcamp is a full, popular class where there's always room for new fitness friends to share the exhilaration of burpee torture with.

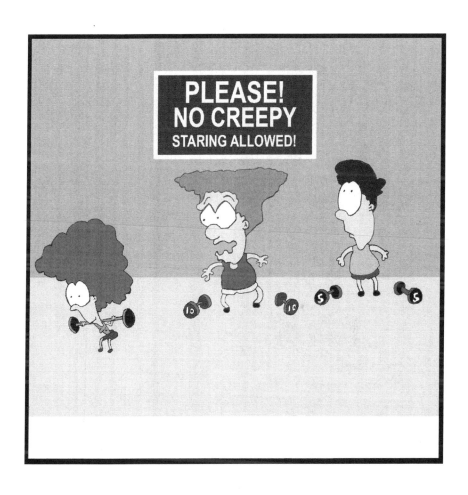

"I walk slowly but I never walk backward."
- Abraham Lincoln

HILDA

I'm very pleased to introduce a very incredible woman and friend of mine. Her name is Hilda and she is a 35-year old, Hispanic woman who is originally from El Paso, Texas. She is happily married and loves Indian food and chocolate. In her spare time, Hilda enjoys reading, making jewelry, and pottery (wheel throwing). After reading her story, it made me realize the reason why I got into teaching in the first place. Although, I don't get tears very often, I definitely did when learning about this woman who I'd see in class. She's always been quiet and has a gentle smile in class and knowing about her and hearing her story makes me very happy that I decided to do this book. I'm very happy to be friends with her and the fact that I get to be one of the characters in her life journey. Thank you so much for sharing your story, I know that it will reach many people and effect so many.

Without further adieu, here's Hilda's story:

I have always had a special love for running. Running was an escape from the alcoholism and drug addiction my brother and I saw on a daily basis, thanks to our uncle. It was an escape from the effects of a mentally ill grandmother who did everything she could to take care of us. It was an escape from the obvious and tangible poverty. Many of my early memories involve my aunt taking me to track meets in Mexico, the place where I was born and raised. I used to run with my older cousins and my brother. We participated in races and I have vivid memories of winning some of these. I remember seeing my name (and sometimes photos) printed in the local newspapers and can still feel the pride I felt then.

Years later, thanks to Reagan's amnesty program and some good luck, my parents were able to migrate to the States. My father had a job, started his own business, and eventually we all moved to El Paso, Texas. The change was extreme, but we managed. Unfortunately, I stopped running and doing any kind of exercise for many years. I started jogging again in my

20s when I was offered a job as a special agent for the FBI, but missed that opportunity because I was unable to pass the physical exam. This, unfortunately, has been one of my biggest regrets. But I think the universe had other plans for me, or at least that is what I choose to believe.

I ran on and off throughout the years, but as tends to happen, I let ____ (insert any of these excuses here: work, school, life, friends, partying, marriage, etc.) take over. In August of 2013, I decided to train for the PF Chang's Rock 'n' Roll half marathon. Life was great! I bought a book that gave me some running tips, a running schedule, and I was finally being consistent with my workouts. During the weekends I would do my long distance running, and during the weekdays I would run and cross train.

Two months later, I felt a lump in my left breast - I made an appointment with my doctor and she assured me that this was nothing to worry about. I was a healthy 33-year old, recently married and hoping to start a family in a year or so. She asked me to keep an eye on this lump, but assured me that it was likely due to monthly hormonal changes. Being the warrior that I am, I begged her for a mammogram consultation. She insisted it was not necessary, but wanted to set my mind was at ease. A month later I got the mammogram. All women over 40 are expected to go through this procedure to make sure there are no signs of breast cancer. For any readers unfamiliar with mammograms, let me attempt to explain what they entail. Women are asked to remove all clothing from the waist up, and given a gown. Then, we are asked to step in front of a strange contraption usually in a cold room, and we are given a list of instructions. The gown is removed, and then a series of mortifying, acrobatic, standing positions follow. Two flat, plastic surfaces painfully compress the breasts, and finally, an x-ray image is taken. Aside from humiliating, the experience is quite nerve-racking. When the radiologist walked over to give me her diagnosis in person, I knew something was wrong. She suggested a biopsy. That was the beginning of the toughest and most enlightening year of my life.

I was diagnosed with invasive adenocarcinoma stage 2b on December 3rd, 2013. The cancer had spread to at least one of my lymph nodes and I needed an oncologist consultation ASAP. That night, my husband and I went to Tempe Beach Park and walked together for a long time. We had recently gotten over his health issues a year previous: now it was my turn. We both nervously cried, then laughed, cried again and discussed our future. We went to bed holding hands praying that this was just a nightmare, but it was not.

During this time, I did the only thing I knew how to do - I ran. I still planned to attempt the half-marathon, but unfortunately the side effects of chemotherapy had different plans for me. My cancer was estrogen-fueled and HER2 positive, and it was suggested that I start four months of chemo right away. During chemo I opted to continue working full-time, and since I was a contractor, my employer was happy to accommodate my schedule. Working full-time was taking a toll on me. In March of 2014, while attempting to ignore the nausea and pain, I went out for a walk/run, and had a seizure in the middle of the street. Thankfully, my husband James was with me, and he was able to handle the situation. This is when I realized I had to stop. I had to learn to listen to my body.

I spent the month of July home, trying to recuperate from a double mastectomy. Running was not an option, but walking felt nice. In September I started a month long radiation treatment. I read an article that recommended patients going through RAD treatments to do a little bit of exercise prior to every session. The exercise was supposed to reduce the effects of fatigue and anemia. In my situation, radiation was a breeze compared to chemo. I woke up every morning and walked for about an hour, went to my treatment, came home and walked a little more. Aside from the skin burns and anxiety from possible future heart issues, etc., life was starting to feel a bit more normal.

The beginning of 2015 was a blur. We weren't sure if we should return to Texas and forget all about Phoenix. I missed my family and wanted to be close to them. I stopped working out and wasn't feeling well. I read that this is normal post-cancer treatments. It was hard to process what cancer did to me; I was now a confused, patchy haired, foggy-minded, scarred and scared woman.

By March I decided to join the gym and take some time off work; a sabbatical if you will. Exercise and time returned some of the self-confidence back. I joined some of the Zumba and BodyWorks classes, which were fun, but a bit unusual for me. Then I came across a bootcamp class one random Thursday morning. The instructor was upbeat and everyone seemed to be enjoying themselves. After attending several bootcamp sessions, I realized how much better I was starting to feel. It wasn't just the exercise; it was the energy in the room, the comradery and the high after each bootcamp. The instructor encouraged the attendees to join him via Facebook to check out bootcamp schedule updates. After a few weeks, I asked him for his Facebook information and with a big smile and sweet disposition, he provided the details. Robby Wagner and I became virtual friends. At the gym, Robby is an instructor that is not afraid to offer feedback and pushes his students to do better by correcting form, or by giving encouraging words. Through Facebook, Robby is a caring, fun, genuine guy that cares about his friends. He is a selfless guy who loves his dog and isn't afraid to take a stand on issues he feels strongly about. Overall, he is a good person to look up to, and someone who is easy to respect.

Bootcamps, running, and sometimes even yoga helped pull me out of a dark place. These have given me back some of my confidence, and needless to say, some of my health. A few months ago, my brother joined one of the free park sessions Robby offers and his class review was hilarious. He could not believe Robby did this for free, and that people do this for fun. His biggest surprise was how much this had changed me from a year ago. I was no longer that frail, bald, sick person everyone saw through photos I sent to my parents letting them know I was still alive. I was a strong, energy filled, unstoppable girl that wanted to hold on to dear life for as long possible. My husband joined the first class offered during Labor Day and his feedback was very similar to my brother's. Why did it feel so good to hear them say that we are all insane and then complain about how sore they were for days? =)

My eating habits have changed. I am back at work. I am working out and life is finally starting to feel normal. I know that due to the surgery my push-ups need a lot of work, but I'll get there. I know I could run faster and for longer periods of time, but I'm working on it. I just picked up my half-marathon training guide. I am hopeful that 2016 will be my half-marathon year. I also know work is important, but not my number one priority. For now, I am happy to be alive and grateful for all of my family and loyal friends who stood by me during the hard times. I am grateful for all the benefits exercise gives me during good and bad days. I am grateful for great leaders and health evangelists, just like Robby, who want to help others without being judgmental and without having ulterior motives. Finally, I am grateful that I was given a second chance to realize how much I love life. Every day is a blessing.

Cool-Down

All my classes end with a proper cool down – and so we will in this book as well. Also like my class, the cool down ends the current workout but not the workout tomorrow or any in the future. After this book, I hope that you discover a purpose for exercise in your life. The stories that you read are not, by any means, an end or a final product of anyone. They are current and will continuously evolve, as fitness is intended to. This continuation will have many ups and downs that are filled with both struggles and accomplishments.

As for myself, I know that this lifestyle is ever growing. I never want to not have something to work toward, learn about, discover about myself, or feel is complete. I've had many highs and lows since my initial weight loss. With the many hurdles life has thrown at me, I've had to find ways to keep going forward – even when I jump and get tripped on the way over them. The key is to not stay down but to learn from the fall and use it as strength to carry on.

With three more challenging weight loss stories since my first one at 18-years old, I've learned that life continuously puts up a great fight against obstacles. And although only temporary, I'm certainly capable of falling off the wagon from time to time. After each time that I've let myself go and then found myself, I've said I'll never get to that point again. I don't see falling off as defeat but as a challenge for me to change again, which I've always been more than willing to accept. I've learned just as much from failing as I have from overcoming such large obstacles. To me, it's not failure at all. Instead, it's a window to understanding my limits, my strengths, my weaknesses, and my character, which always fights to be better.

I really hope you enjoyed <u>My Burpee's Shadow</u> and found some inspiration to help you begin your own journey into this unending and, in my opinion, undefinable wide world of heath and fitness. It's most certainly not easy to start but very exciting one once you get going. I've never met a single person who didn't say that it is more difficult to stop than it is to continue. I hope that you fall in love with exercise and all of the other wonderful things that it leads to: nutrition, energy,

happiness, creativity, perspective on life, love, and overall wellness. Your story, like everyone's in this book, is unique and special. Take advantage of it. Embrace it. And no matter what, always strive to be better each day and never let anything get in the way of you and your health!

Connect with me at:

www.robbywagner.com